The Herbal Apprentice Work Book

Abrah Arneson Cht. RH

ISBN:0993906923
ISBN-13:9780993906923

To my Mom

Being rock, being gas, being mist, being Mind,
Being the mesons traveling amongst galaxies with the speed of light,
You have come here, my beloved…
You have manifested yourself as trees, as grass, as
Butterflies, as single –cell beings, and as
chrysanthemums;
but the eyes with which you looked at me this morning
tell me you have never died. – Thich Nhat Hanh

Contents

Working with plant medicine is a complex dance. There is the dance between the herbalist and the plant, the plant and person using the medicine, and the herbalist and person taking the medicine. Ultimately though, plant medicine is the profoundly intricate and often mysterious dance of the inter-being between all life on this beautiful planet.

The Herbal Apprentice Work Book, along with its accompanying book *The Herbal Apprentice: Plant Medicine and The Human Being*, is written to support you in developing confidence to step into the elegant dance between plant medicine and the human being.

There was a time when herbalists used dreams and meditation to intuit a plant's medicine and the nature of the health challenge to be healed. In this work book, I am attempting to wake up these traditional ways of using plant medicine without throwing out the analytical scientific knowledge of our time. It is my intention that by combining these approaches you will be able to quickly learn your own unique steps in the dance between plant medicine and the human being.

In this work book you will find techniques and exercises to deepen your understanding of the healing nature of meditation and dreams while delving into practical lessons in herbal medicine and medicine making. This work book takes you on a personal healing journey, enhancing your confidence and gifts as a healer while enriching your first-hand knowledge of plant medicine.

I would like to thank all the herbal apprentices I have worked with over the years — you have all been my teachers. Thank you for the laughter, the tears and sharing the joy of plant medicine.

Thank you to both Dionne Jennings and Trudy Gold for their patient editing of this work book. Dionne also gave me the great photograph on the cover of this book. The photograph features Lindsey, Lu, Jen, Dani, Krysta and Tanya garbling Mugwort in Lindsey's yurt resting in the magnificent Rocky Mountain foothills. Thank you all for offering your beauty for the cover of this book.

I would like to thank all the clients I have worked with over the years. Without your trust in this very old medicine, I don't know where I would be today. Thank you choosing sustainable medicine.

I extend heartfelt gratitude all plants for giving themselves freely. From my green friends I learn so much about being human, living in community and healing. It is my wish that you, dear reader, discover faith in the goodness of all life on this planet through the use of plant medicine.

Stay green,

Abrah

How to Use this Work Book

This work book is an accompaniment to The Herbal Apprentice: Plant Medicine and The Human Being. It is for those who wish to drink deeply from the roots of plant medicine and learn to think like a herbalist.

Within the first couple of months of opening my clinical practice, a woman asked me to accept her as an apprentice. Having just graduated from The Dominion Herbal Colleges Clinical Herbal Therapist program, I turned her down. How could I teach what I was still learning?

A couple of months later, a man made the same request. I also turned him down. Within six months of opening my clinic, five people asked if they could apprentice under me.

Finally I thought, "Well I can try." That thought was the beginning of The Herbal Apprentice and this work book.

The lessons in this work book have been crafted over a period of years as more and more people arrived at my door to learn about herbal medicine. It is my intention that this work book will help you to discover your inner herbalist.

What do I mean by that?

Every herbalist I know who practices herbal medicine has uncovered their own unique way of using plant medicine to help others. There is certainly essential knowledge a herbalist needs, but how this knowledge translates into her methods of helping others with plant medicine is unique.

Herbalists are a combination of their individual life experiences, beliefs, gifts, weaknesses and communication styles. The plants growing near the herbalist's home support their understanding of plant medicine. The community the herbalist serves guides the herbalist in their discovering new or old ways of using plant medicine. Ultimately each student of herbal medicine learns to think like an herbalist.

The lessons in this work book are crafted to help you learn to think like an herbalist while drawing from your own life experiences, beliefs, gifts, weaknesses and communication styles. The lessons in this book will send you out to explore the plants in your neighbourhood (all neighbourhoods have plants). It is my hope that with this work book you develop the confidence to learn from the teachers of herbal medicine: the plants themselves.

What you will need

To begin you will need three notebooks. One to record your journey as a healer. Call this notebook your Healing Journal. This notebook will include your dreams, visions, challenges, inspirations, etc.

In a second notebook you will record your medicine making experiences. Call this one your Medicine Making Notebook.

Finally, in the third notebook you will write down your findings as you discover plants. It is for teachings specifically on plants. You can call this notebook whatever you like.

For the medicine making book and the plant book I recommend binders. You can easily add information as you go with a binder. You can also use different types of paper to record information. You may want to include drawings or photographs using blank paper while you record with the written word on lined paper. (As you can see, I am old school. Still lugging around books, binders, and notebooks. If you feel good managing all the information you will gather on your computer or another devise, then please use what you are most comfortable with.)

There are number of books I recommend you get from the library or purchase for your own healing library. They are listed in Appendix 1 at the back of the work book. Each of these books I have found useful in my journey as herbalist and healer.

You will also need to find a place where you can purchase dried herbs. Most cities have herb shops. If you live in a town or out in the country where there is no herb shop I recommend you seek out a reliable supplier of dried, ethically harvested, sustainable, high-grade plant medicine.

You will need the willingness to discover who you are as a herbalist and healer as well as welcome mistakes as an opportunity to learn. You need to keep an open mind.

Appendix 2 lists the herbs and other medicine making supplies you will need for each lesson.

Exploring the Lessons

Each lesson broken into ten sections. The sections are:

1. Healer Heal Thyself
2. Meditation
3. Reflections
4. Understanding Body/Mind
5. Creative Monographs
6. Enhanced Herbal Knowledge
7. Medicine Making
8. Dreams

Sometimes I find students excel in one section, put in their time with other sections and then leave a section out. Usually the section or exercises students avoid are uncomfortable for them. The section challenges their weakness.

I strongly recommend you do your best with each section. Try everything. Do not grade yourself, criticize yourself or think your experience with each lesson or section should be different then it is. Make your learning experience your own. Let the lessons reveal your gifts and weaknesses. Let them teach you how you learn best. Let the lessons uncover your inner healer and herbalist.

Section One

Healer Heal Thyself

It is well known that a healer can only help others where she has been wounded and is healing. (Notice I said healing not healed. Healing is a journey not a singular event.) The explorations in this section will take you on a healing journey, challenging your limitation, discovering your gifts and enhancing your self-awareness. Infuse yourself with these exercise. They will sooth your wounds and bring compassion into your heart for the most important person in your life — you. Once you offer yourself with compassion, it is not difficult to walk in compassion for the rest of life on this beautiful planet.

Some of the exercises in this section are difficult. Do the best you can with them. It is possible to always return to them later when you feel ready to explore those parts of yourself you have not yet ready to touched.

Section Two

Meditation

You may be a seasoned meditator or someone who believes they are incapable of meditation. In either case, throw out everything you think you know about meditation and give yourself the chance to try the meditations in this work book like a beginner.

In my personal healing journey, meditation is one of my greatest tools. It helps me remain honest, grounded and open to life. Being a healer is not always easy. Healers witness many sorrows and much pain. In my experience, meditation is the medicine that allows you to stay open, not walk away carrying another's pain nor turn away from another's sorrow. Meditation guides you in the honesty needed to help others.

Each lesson offers a different meditation. Try each one for a week, taking about 10 to 20 minutes a day. Notice how it affects you. If you like its effects carry on with the meditation. If you do not notice any change, try another one. If you are curious about another meditation, explore it.

The most important advice I can offer, after having practiced meditation for 30 years is this: never think you know how to meditate and never believe you cannot meditate. Let meditation meditate you!

Section Three

Reflections

The reflections are a series of quotes that are designed to inspire you, challenge you and give you something to think about. Some may strike a chord and others may feel like a splinter. I suggest you begin each day with three repetitions of the reflections and let them steep into your being.

Section Four

Understanding Body/Mind

This section explores the human being's wondrous body and mind with the intention of broadening both your knowledge, appreciation and understanding for the life it contains.

Section Five

Creative Monographs

When I first started to teach herbal medicine I gave my apprentices a form outlining the orthodox method of recording information on healing plants. The form was called a monograph. Oh! the grief my apprentices gave me about this form. They lamented that the monographs were tedious, difficult to remember and stressing them out! Personally I find stress and learning are not happy companions so I came up with "creative Monographs".

A creative monograph includes all the information an orthodox monograph includes, but it is done with a creative flare in a manner the apprentice will most likely recall.

I have had students sing creative monographs, paint creative monographs, create collages of plant monographs, crossword puzzles and word finds, write stories and poems, draw comic strips, and many other methods of building a plant monograph to suit their personal talent and learning style. The most important aspect of compiling a creative monograph is to not take it too seriously and let yourself play.

Below is an example of an orthodox monograph. I strongly suggest you include the headings found in this monograph in some way with your creative monograph. Also if you want to create orthodox monographs because that method suits you best, please do.

Example of Orthodox Monograph

Mentha piperita
Common Name: Peppermint, Black Mint
Family: Labiatae
Keynote: Antispasmodic, digestive tonic. Used in nausea, flatulence and dyspepsia, carminative.
Parts used and Harvest: Herb and distilled oil, herb, harvest before flowering

Character or energetics: Pungent, dry, generally cooling
Systems: Nerves, gastro-intestinal
Constituents: Essential oils, Flavonoids, Rosmarinic acid, azulenes, choline, carotenes
Actions: Spasmolytic, carminative, anti-emetic, diaphoretic, anti-septic, anti-viral, peripheral vasodilation, emmenagogue, source for potassium and magnesium, enzyme activator, cooling, cholagogue, analgesic, digestive tonic, nervine, aromatic
Indications:

> Herbal tea blends for indigestion, colic, cough, and cold
> Excess mucous secretion
> Relaxes muscles of digestive tract, Stimulates bile flow
> Motion sickness and nausea, mild anaesthetic on the stomach wall
> Ulcerative colitis and crohn's
> Flues and fever
> Migraine headache associated with digestion
> Eases anxiety, tension, hysteria, infant convulsions
> Gall bladder disease

Essential oil   Analgesic, calming

> Skin complaints
> Fevers
> Headaches and migraines linked to over heating
> Anti-bacterial, clears nasal congestion
> Insect repellent
> Raises depressed spirits
> Infant convulsions

Compress   Inflamed joints, rheumatism and neuralgia
Massage oil   Relieve congestion during breast feeding, menstrual pain
Combinations:

> Colds and flues: Boneset, Peppermint, Elderflowers, Yarrow

Preparations:

> Infusion: 102 tsp dried herb in 1 cup boiling water. Infuse 5-10 minutes. Drink freely.
> Tincture: 1:5 in 45% alcohol. Dose: 2-4 ml
> > Concentrated peppermint oil: 1 part peppermint oil in 30 parts 90% alcohol. Add gradually, with repeated shaking. 50 parts distilled oil. 5-20 drops freely.
> Powder: 2-4 grams

Massage oil: 5-6 drops in almond or olive oil for cramps, spasms, lower back ache, sports injuries, stiffness of shoulders and joints.

Contra-indicated and Cautions:

Pregnancy, anxiety neurosis, nervous excitability

Other Herbal Systems:

Folklore: In India they say, "If one can name all the actions of peppermint on the human body, one can name all the fish in the Indian Ocean."

Example of Creative Monograph

Blue Cohosh

They,
people who walked barefoot and were not afraid of the dark,
found stories everywhere.

Strawberry, for instance,
grew on Star Woman's daughter's grave.

Star Woman, by the way, fell
through a hole in the sky
and then danced
till her feet were muddy again.

Grass used to be the earth's hair.
Corn, beans and squash were sisters.
Mushrooms were doctors.
Apples offered offending knowledge.

The trembling aspen's down fall was pride.
Birch was the Lady of the Forest.
Lonely trees in fields were homes of lost souls.

Stories used to be everywhere. Everything spoke.

Let me tell you a well-known secret.
I walk in bare feet and am not afraid of the dark.
When I am in the mood to listen,
everywhere I hear a story.

Yesterday, wearing my hiking boots, a story found me.

I brushed away the crumbled leaves and loose soil –

first to appear were four hard shoots
like bruised nipples, obviously -
she had prepared for spring.

With my digging stick,
I dug deeper.

Her roots did not wander,
nor did they branch.
They were thin and course
like thick black hair bleached white.
They burrowed into the forest soil,
clinging to the dark, damp clumps.
As if life depended on it.

The roots descended from a gnarled rhizome.
curling into itself like a grief struck woman.

I gently gathered the roots in my hands.
And lifted her from her bed.
My stomach hollowed out.
The way it does when I see a sick baby,
tubes in his nose, skin fire red, in a plastic box.
Mum wearing a mask.

Still on my knees,
I hold the roots to my face.
Breathe deeply.
Sweet, soft, sour.
Like hope turned to despair.

Washing away the soil was uncomfortable
as exposing another's labia to the light of day.

Once the forest told me to sing.
"Only hunters walk in silence", the trees whispered.

So I sang to the roots.
Easing the fear, the loss.
Letting her know I heard her sorrow.

If I could tell her story it would go something like this:
There is a plant that grows for every woman who tried to give it birth
to the child who refuses to be born.

Now she sits in a jar, in the kitchen,
waiting to be medicine.   - Abrah Arneson

Section Six

Enhanced Herbal Knowledge

This section delves deeper into plant medicine. Usually it involves
different traditions or more technical aspects of plant medicine.

Section Seven

Medicine Making

All the apprentices I have ever worked with want to make plant
medicine. Medicine making is hands on and practical. In this section we
create many different types of plant medicine. Follow along with the
recipes and guidelines on making medicine, but also use your common
sense so if something does not seem right — change it up and see what
happens. Most of the best medicine I have ever made came about
because of a blend of tradition, mistakes, using what I had on hand,
beautiful plants and a little prayer.

To get the most out of your medicine making I strongly recommend you
keep good notes in your Medicine Making Notebook. By using my
notebook and referring back to it, I have learned from my mistakes and
replicated my triumphs. In the chart below are a few things you may
want to record. You may copy the chart into your notebook or develop
your own method for recording your plant medicine.

Date	Plant	Method	Results	Notes
Rose Hip Syrup 9/10/15	Fresh Rosehips	400 grams rose hips (fresh), 800 ml of water, 1 c. honey Simmer to tender. Mash. Simmer 8 mins. Pour into cheesecloth, drip overnight. Pressed. Return to saucepan, add honey, blend. Refrigerate.	Yummy dense syrup But went off in 6 weeks when not put in the fridge.	Wild crafted hips after 1st killing frost. Easier to way to separate out seeds?

Section Eight

Dreams

From the very beginning herbalists have dreamt of plants and their medicine. I strongly recommend you use this work book to begin or deepen your journey as a dreamer.

Section Nine

Other Resources

In this section I recommend you seek out videos found on the internet to enhance your learning. There are lots of great videos that gently explain the anatomy and physiology of the body as well as medicine making techniques. It is good to hear what other herbalists have to say about different herbs, health challenges and medicine making techniques. I will also you purchase the books in the reading list to refer to while exploring the topics in this work book. I have found all these books quite useful. books are listed in Appendix 3.

One final word

Enjoy your discovery of the wonderful world of plant medicine and the human being.

Lesson One
It's All About the Environment

Please read chapter one in The Herbal Apprentice: Plant Medicine and The Human Being.

Healer Heal Thyself

What is your relationship with colours and the elements?

Humans have a powerful relationship to colour. We have favourite colours. We dislike colours. We use colour to express love. We decorate our homes with specific colours at celebratory times of the year. Colour is used to suggest caution, to give us the go ahead and to stop our forward momentum. Sometimes a colour can even fill hearts with hatred. Whether we like or dislike a colour is generally to do with the memories the colour evokes and the accompanying emotions.

Mostly we are not aware of the emotions and memory colours evoke. Our talking minds override these subtle details with stories about the colour such as, "Blue is my favourite colour because it is calm and expansive like the sky or sea," or, "I strongly dislike green pants with pockets on the thighs, it reminds me of war."

I will share with you an experience I have had with the bold colours red, yellow and orange.

I am a child of the sixties. After the conforming greys and soft blues of the fifties, the sixties exploded into big colours: orange, red, purple! These vibrant non-conforming colours burst out all over. I remember the fabric on airplane seats covered in bright orange flowers with a red and purple background. Could you image that today?

My parents had four children and I was the only female child. My brothers shared a room and I had my own. My room was the smallest in the house and its walls were covered in wallpaper splashed with a cacophony of huge red, orange and yellow flowers. The brightness and size of the colours were overwhelming to my child's mind. I also felt alone in my room, listening to my brothers' talk and laugh on the other side of the wall.

I have a complex relationship with these colours. I can only take them in small doses now. I feel too big if I wear all red, too loud in orange and I avoid yellow all together. When I enter a room that is dominated in any of these colours, or meet someone dressed only in one of the these colours, I find I become quiet inside and a little shy. In the large presence of these colours I need time to feel centered.

It is very important as a healer to understand the personal meanings and memories you associate with each colour. You will respond to people who wear your favourite colour in a different manner than those wearing a colour that triggers you. As a healer, by learning to appreciate different colours you will become more flexible in your ability to appreciate the people around you and the environment that contains you. You will also learn a lot about your clients by the colours they choose to wear and surround themselves in.

To take our exploration of colour a little further, each element has a colour. The colours vary from tradition to tradition. It is not that a particular tradition has the right set of colours for the elements. I think it is a matter of the environment that tradition evolved in, the perception of the people practicing the tradition and their relationship with the element and the element's assigned colour.

Because most of my training in working with the elements and colour comes from the Buddhist tradition, we will work with the colours assigned to the elements in that tradition. If you have a strong affinity with another tradition or are exploring the rituals and ceremonies from another tradition you are welcome to explore those colours of the elements.

Here is how colours and elements are paired in the Buddhist tradition.

Earth	Yellow
Water	Sky blue (sometimes white)
Fire	Red
Air	Green
Space	White (sometimes dark blue)

Colours like orange are a blend of earth and fire element while purple is fire and water mingling.

Try this...

For a couple of days, wear only your favourite colour. Notice how you feel in this colour and how people respond to you. You will probably not notice much as this is your "normal." Also notice how you respond to people wearing your favourite colour.

For a couple of days, wear a colour that you dislike. It does not have to be your whole outfit, perhaps a scarf, vest, t-shirt. Notice how you feel in this colour and how people respond to you. People will respond in a different manner depending on their relationship to the colour. Notice how you respond to people wearing this colour.

Then for a day wear black as the dominant colour.

The next day wear white as the dominant colour.

Pick a day to wear red as the primary colour of your clothing.

The next day, wear blue.

Then go on to explore other colours that evoke a strong feeling and those that don't.

Write down your observations of, feelings about and response to each colour. Notice if you can see a relationship between the dominant element in a person and their choices of colour. Review the characteristics of the different elements: their physical, emotional and spiritual manifestation as noted by traditional herbalists in *The Herbal Apprentice: Plant Medicine and The Human Being.*

Meditation

Then tell me, what is the material world, and is it dead?
He laughing answer'd: I will write a book on leaves of flowers,
If you will feed me on loving-thoughts, & give me now and then
A cup of sparkling poetic fancies: so when I am tipsie,
I'll sing to you to this soft lute; and shew you all alive
The world, every particle of dust breathes forth its joy.
From Europe a Prophecy by William Blake

Nature is alive. Human beings, mind, body and spirit are part of nature. Plants — trees, grasses, berries, flowers, prickly cacti — are alive. Rocks are alive. Soil is a living ecology of bacteria, fungi, worms and mycelium.

Air is alive with viruses, yeasts and bacteria. This world, even the world you cannot see, hear, smell, touch or taste, is alive.

Let's begin with cultivating an understanding of this boundless livingness with meditation on Loving kindness.

Lovingkindness is a beautiful practice to do before falling asleep (you can do it laying in your bed while falling asleep) or walking in a city, forest, town or meadow. It can also be done as a more formal practice. By this I mean meditating for a specific time period at a certain time of day.

For example: I consider my formal practice to be what I do between 7:00 and 8:00 am on most days. My informal practice is while I walk Bubbaloo, my black lab, stand in line at the grocery store, cook dinner or do dishes, etc.

Because lovingkindness is closely associated with a sensual experience of beauty, one begins the practice with a creative visualization of beauty.

The Heart Center is also referred to as the heart chakra. It is the heart of your energy body. When you connect with your heart center, there is willing receptivity to the world. The heart center is a patient place that allows life to happen on its own time and you to receive the moment. The heart center is located just in front of your spine in the center of your chest.

During every day there are beautiful moments. It may be when you first wake and soft sunlight fills your bedroom. Or it may be on your drive home from work while the setting sun illuminates clouds with orange and red light. Perhaps your child's smile ignites beauty in your heart. There are innumerable manifestations of beauty in the world. Which are most meaningful to you?

To begin:

Gently bring forth a memory of beauty. Try to pick a memory of a "normal" type of beauty. A beauty you experience every day. To pull the memory into this moment and evoke the experience of beauty ask yourself the following questions:

❖ Where were you?
❖ What did you see, hear, small or taste during this memory of beauty?
❖ Who were you with?

When you feel that you have recreated the memory of beauty, begin to gently breath into your heart center.

The experience of beauty creates a soft openness in your heart center. When you get really good at invoking beauty you will have an experience of warmth spreading from your heart center into the rest of your body. It is blissful. This warm, soft openness is how your body/mind experiences lovingkindness.

Once you have the feeling of beauty in your heart, think or say out loud the following words:

May I be happy and fully satisfied.
May I be free of anxiety, disease and anger.
May I guard myself with happiness.   *(repeat 3 times)*
As you say this, image the feeling of lovingkindness spreads through your body.

Next image all the human beings you know and think:

May all human beings I know be happy and fully satisfied

May they be free of anxiety, disease and anger.
May they guard themselves with happiness.   *(repeat 3 times)*
As you say this, image the feeling of lovingkindness spreads through your body and out to all the human beings you know.

Then repeat the meditation while considering all the human beings you don't know. Feel your experience of lovingkindness spread out to all the human beings you do not know.

Next, offer lovingkindness to all the mammals you know.

Then offer lovingkindness to all the mammals you do not know.

Continue the meditation offering lovingkindness to each of the following:

All fish you know.   All fish you do not know.

All birds you know.   All birds you do not know.

All reptiles you know.   All reptiles you do not know.

All amphibians you know.   All amphibians you do not know.

All crustaceans you know.   All crustaceans you do not know.

All insects you know.   All insects you do not know.

All arachnidan you know   All the arachnidan you not know

All trees you know.   All trees you do not know.

All herbaceous plants you know. All herbaceous plants you do not know.

All cacti you know.   All cacti you do not know.

All fungi you know.   All fungi you do not know.

All lichen you know.   All lichen you do not know.

All seaweeds you know. All seaweeds you do not know.

All algae you know.   All algae you do not know.

All rocks you know.   All rocks you do not know.

All angels you know.   All angels you do not know.

Finish with yourself:

May I be happy and fully satisfied
May I be free of all anxiety, disease and anger.
May I guard myself with happiness.
By practicing lovingkindness in this way over a period of several months, you will develop a sense of the livingness of all plants, mushrooms and animals on our beautiful plants. You will discover the beauty in all of creation and understand how each living being cherishes its precious life. Lovingkindness brings great healing to all life.

Another way of doing this practice is wishing lovingkindness for every living being you encounter during the day. This can be done by mentally saying:
May you be happy and fully satisfied.

Reflection

Hippocrates said, "Where ever the art of medicine is practiced, there is a love of humanity."

Write a paragraph or two about how you love humanity. Repeat Hippocrates quote three times each morning to yourself for a couple of weeks.

Understanding the Body/Mind

In the spiritual tradition that I study, Tibetan Buddhism, the elements earth, water, fire, air and space are not alive. For the elements to become alive, they must be mingled with consciousness. The elements give structure to conscious.

In Tibetan Buddhism it is said, "Consciousness, which has eyes but no legs, rides a horse that has legs but no eyes." The horse represents the elements. The eyes represent consciousness.

The elements mix and mingle to create the myriad forms of the universe. Consciousness embodies the myriad of forms the elements create. It is important to understand that the elements and their many combinations affects the consciousness embodied within the formations they create as much as consciousness affects the form (the elements) it animates.

Let's begin with a study of the elements and their relationship to consciousness. To understand how the elements and consciousness

---

If you are thinking, "What is she going on about?" Try to think of consciousness and the elements in this way:

Let's say consciousness is like water. Water takes on the form of the vessel it is poured into. The vessel represents the other elements. The shape of the vessel affects how the water pours, the temperature of the water, perhaps even the colour and the contents of the water. When the vessel breaks (as elements do eventually break up, usually called death) the water flows out of it and takes on a new shape. This is an example of how the elements (the vessel) and consciousness (the water) interact.

---

interact, you will use yourself as a laboratory.

Healing Journal Activity

Consider these questions for one month and make notes in your Healing Journal.

❖ How do different manifestations of the elements attract or repel you?

To observe the fire element and consider these questions:

❖ How does your body respond to cold and warmth? How does your mind respond to different temperatures? Can you change how your mind reacts to heat or cold? Can you change your body's reaction?

❖ Notice how others respond to warmth and cold? How do their body types and mind differ from each other and yourself?

❖ What have you learned about the fire element in your observations?

To observe the air (or wind) element and ask:

❖ How does your body respond to windy days and calm days? How does your mind react to wind? Is it the same as on calm days? Can you change your mind's or body's reaction?

❖ Stop several times a day and notice three breaths without changing them. How do you breathe differently throughout the day?

❖ Notice how others respond to wind? How do their body types and mind differ from each other and yourself?

❖ What have you learned about the wind element in your observations?

To observe the water element and consider the following questions:

❖ What is your relationship with water?

❖ Pay attention to water, thank the water when you bath, cook or drink it. Talk to the water. Listen to water.

❖ Go for a morning or afternoon without using water.

❖ What have you learned about the water element in your observations?

To observe the earth element, try the following exercises.

❖ When you eat food, think of yourself as eating earth. Thank the earth. Can you feel the presence of earth in your body?

❖ Take a walk and pay attention to the earth under your feet. Notice how it continually unfolds before you. (This experience is quite powerful when you have hiked up a mountain trail to a grand vista.) As you walk, quietly say to yourself, earth. What do you notice?

❖ Lay down under a tree. Then lay down in an open area. Next lay (or sit) on cement. Walk barefoot in mud. How do experience the earth in each place?

❖ What have you learned about the earth element in your observations?

Creative Monographs

With a playful heart create a monograph for each element: earth, water, fire, air and space.

Enhancing Herbal Knowledge

Go for a walk in landscapes dominated by an element. For example: rocky landscapes have a dominant earth element, swamps and sloughs are water, open spaces may have dominant air, dry places are powerfully affected by the heat of the sun or the fire element. Notice the type of plants that grow there. What is common about the plants in these environments? What types of adaptation have they made? Compare the nature of the plants growing in each landscape.

Notice how the elements affect each other in the different landscapes. How does water, fire, air change the quality of the earth element? How does a lack of fire element alter the other elements? What is the relationship of water to the other elements? How does the wind play in or destroy a landscape?

Medicine Making

Making a Medicine Bag

Herbalists often carry a small medicine bag with them when they practice their art. The medicine bag contains plants and prayers that they believe will help them stay true to their plants, their profession, their clients and the living spirit of this beautiful planet.

Make your medicine bag. You may choose any type of cloth or animal skin. Even if you have no skill with needle and thread, try to create your own. While you are stitching together your medicine bag, consider how you want to honour the living spirit of plants, animals, humans and this beautiful planet.

Then find yourself some hawthorn berries. Discover why I recommend the medicine from the wise and honest hawthorn tree. Hint: go back in time to stories from the Celts.

Place the hawthorn berries in your medicine bag. Write a prayer or song for the hawthorn and put it in your medicine bag as well. You may want to add another plant that you feel teaches you to the medicine bag. In mine, I have a bear's tooth, as the bear is an animal I have had many encounters with and feel guides me on my journey as a healer.

Rose Hip Syrup

This is your first wild crafting adventure. First Nations people say that it is necessary to have your mind in a good way to pick medicine. When you go out to wild craft, go joyfully. Try not to pick a day when you have many tasks to accomplish. Give yourself precious time.

> Garbling happens after you have picked your medicine from the wild or your garden. Garbling is carefully looking over the plants and removing any unhappy looking parts. Perhaps you discover a partially eaten hip, or a leaf with eggs laid on it, or lower parts that look like it has been peed on by a dog. All these you remove so they do not make their way into the medicine.

Sometimes when I pick medicine I notice a feeling overtakes me. I often find that the feeling is either the healing the plant offers, or if it is an unpleasant feeling, it is what the plant heals. Pay attention when picking your plants. Stay present. Be aware also of the insects you are interacting with, other animals, plants and weather.

Most berries and hips made by rose family plants are gathered for medicine after the first killing frost. (You may want to discover why.) Therefore, the morning the ground is covered white water crystals (notice the change in the air, water and fire element) go out and pick your hips or hawthorn berries.

Please read the notes below on wild crafting below before going out to pick the rose hips.

Recipe

400 grams rose hips (ripe)

800 ml of water (distilled)

1 cup honey

Instructions:

❖ Gather your hips.

❖ Garble the hips.

❖ Using a stainless steel or enamel saucepan, simmer the dried hips for 15 minutes or until tender. (With fresh hips, this part can be omitted; one can go straight to mashing).

❖ Mash with a wooden spoon. Simmer another 8 minutes.

❖ Pour into several layers of cheesecloth and allow the mashed hips to drip overnight into ceramic bowl. In the morning, squeeze out what remains in the cheese cloth.

❖ Return the juice to saucepan, add honey, and stir. Gently melt honey without boiling the hips. Pour into jars and label.

❖ Store in the refrigerator.

Jot down a few ways you would use the syrup. How would you dose it?

If you do not live in an area where you can pick rose hips, substitute the rosehip for elderberries which you can purchase at any good apothecary or on-line.

Guidelines for wild crafting...

1. Ask the plant for permission to gather it. Give thanks and acknowledge the connection between all of life while making an offering to the plant. You can offer a stand of your hair, a pinch of tobacco, a little water, a breath...

2. When you see the first plant you intend to pick as medicine, walk by it while acknowledging its presence. Do this with the next six plants you see. You will walk by a total of seven plants. These are the ancestor plants.

For example, if you are looking for wild rose plants to pick rose hips and come upon a rose plant, with hips drooping from its prickly twigs, acknowledge it and walk by. Walk by six more and then begin to pick when you arrive at the next stand.

Never pick from the last plant you see.

3. Do not pick the roots of an endangered or threatened species. Always be sure you leave the plant with the opportunity to reproduce.

4. Leave most mature plants. These are called Grandparent plants. This is really important if you are picking roots.

5. Seeds run downhill, if harvesting on a slope, work your way up.

6. Harvest no more than 20% from the plants and gather only in abundant plant stands. Check your desire for more or your anxiety that you do not have enough.

7. Use gardening techniques: root division, thinning, and top pinching. It is best to study the area you want to pick in to understand the relationship between the plants you want to pick, other plants that grow in their community and animals who use the plants for food, shelter and protection. Particularly be aware of insects when you are picking. (Often it is best to study an area where medicine grows for a year to become familiar with its ways before gathering medicine. I like to think of this as a time of courtship — becoming intimate with the plants, animals, soil, water, etc. that mix to create the medicine in the plant.

8. When picking leaves, be gentle so the roots stay in the earth.

9. After digging roots, scatter the seeds of the plant and carefully replace the dirt you have removed. If possible, avoid using shovels and take the time a trowel requires to dig roots. You will have a more intimate experience of the plant and its surroundings. Trowels create less disturbance to the earth and the area the plant grows in.

10. Know the plant you want to pick. Be sure! In Canada, I prefer the Lone Pine series of books for plant identification.

11. If wild crafting on public or private land, ask permission

12. Stay away from down-wind pollution, roadsides, high-tension electric wires, public parks and areas where there has been heavy fertilization or pesticide/herbicide use.

Dreams:

Watch how the elements manifest themselves in your dreams. For example:

What kind of floors are you standing on in your dreams? Or what types of natural landscapes do you find yourself in and how are the elements interacting in your dream?

Ask for a dream about the element you are most curious about and the one that you are most uncomfortable about.

Try to catch your dreams and write them down in your journal.

Lesson Two

Beginning at the Beginning: Sensing

Please read chapter two in The Herbal Apprentice: Plant Medicine and The Human Being.

Healer Heal Thyself

Healing is a journey of transformation. Healing is the process of changing from one condition into another. It is alchemical. Healing carries mystery with it. Healing is an act of faith: a willingness to receive the unknown moment and its gifts. Healing has a kind of grace about it.

My Aunt had a grand love affair with her second husband. He took her on adventures around the world that she had never dreamt of. He gave her his joy of nature. I remember being awestruck by a small clearing of wild violets sheltered by a ring of maples one spring. She took me to this beautiful place that he had shown her. She in turn gentled him. Gave him the comforts of a home. Taught him to cook. Unfortunately, they both had a thirst for alcohol.

Alcohol changed their love into a hunger that was a bottomless pit. They tore their love apart with hungry words. The marriage ended.

Years later my aunt was diagnosed with stage four stomach cancer. She died 6 months later. Four month before she died, he arrived at her door. Hundreds of miles away, he had by chance been in the same restaurant as my uncle who was on holidays.

The last four months of my aunt's life was spent with her ex-husband. He cooked for her, bathed her, warmed her blankets, held her and read to her. In illness their hungry words fell away, and gentleness returned to their love. The bitterness and anger they carried fell away. A healing occurred. When she died, she became another defeated statistic in the

24

fight against cancer. Although there was no cure, a healing had occurred.

Healing is like a thread that weaves us whole. The gifts of the plant medicine, the wholeness of the person seeking healing and the healer's ability to be present for the healing bring livingness to the thread. The healing thread over time weaves resolution and newness for every person (and I suspect every plant) touched by the alchemy of the journey.

Considering the numerous synchronicities that occur to create the right alchemy for a healing to take place makes my mind turns to the conversation between the chemist and shaman deep in the amazon forest.

The shaman explains the plant medicine and the chemist takes notes and a sample of the plant. Then the shaman says, "But it is only when the energy of the healer is present that the plant heals." Or at least that is what the chemist hears as it is he who tells us the story.

I suspect the shaman was trying to tell the chemist something quite different. Having worked with plant medicine for some time I have noticed the more I ask the medicine to help me, the more profound the healing and transformation. I have also noticed the more faith the person taking the medicine has, the deeper the healing. I have watched many lives transform over a period of several days, months, and years while healing is taking place.

When involved in a healing I experience the healing thread weaving us, the plant medicine, the person seeking healing and me the healer, together. I have often felt the healing thread has a life, an intelligence of its own. The thread over time stitches together a new life for all of us. Just as the person who is being healed changes, so does the healer. It is impossible to participate in healing and not be transformed in some way.

I suspect this is true for the plant as well. Indigenousness people say that if a plant's medicine is not regularly used with respect and gratitude, the plant goes away. Perhaps somehow the plant's spirit, as it dances between the healer and the one seeking healing, is also transformed.

If it is true that the healing thread weaves its power of transformation between the plant, the healer and the one seeking healing, then the healer needs to let go as much as her client does. She needs to change as the plant does.

Let's for a moment go back to the word "gifts." Remember a couple paragraphs back: "The gifts of the plant medicine, the wholeness of the person seeking healing and the healer's ability to be present brings a livingness to the healing thread." The healer's gifts twist the individual fibers of the healing thread, making it strong.

When a healer sits with confidence in her gifts, healing will take place. When she is able to evoke the gifts of the person seeking healing, there is an even greater possibility that the healing will take place. When she has appreciation and gratitude for the gifts of healing plants, I am certain a healing will take place.

We heal from our gifts. It is our weaknesses, sorrows, fears, anger and illnesses that are healed. Our gifts do the work of healing.

So often when healing is needed we turn our focus on the challenges we are struggling with and try to fix them. When what we need to do is discover our gifts and offer them to the challenges we face. It is our gifts that open us to the grace of healing.

In this lesson, let's explore your gifts.

Gifts are not talents. Talents are things you can do well, like cooking, singing, gardening, etc. Gifts are much more intangible. Gifts are qualities or even more vague, feeling tones. Our gifts are so familiar to us that they are almost impossible to realize. Understanding your gifts is like fish knowing the water they swim in, or humans noticing the air they are breathing. This is how gifts are.

To begin understanding your gifts think about times during the day when you are content. Happy. Peaceful. Joyful. Curious. Playful. If you can't think of a time like this during your day, then set an intention to discover these feelings during the day. Perhaps you will notice contentment when you are driving on a country road singing to a song on the radio while your eyes dance across the open landscape. Perhaps you feel playful as your child's face becomes animated with a funny story about school. Find the moment of these feelings during your day. These feelings are pleasurable.

Once you have found the moment of pleasure, ask: what am I bringing to this moment? What you bring to those moments are your gifts.

In Your Healing Journal

Begin to explore different types of moments during the day when you feel present. When you are just being you. Moments when you are not planning the next moment or fretting about a past moment, just being here now. I promise you there are many of these moments in your day; you just need to practice noticing them.

You may find yourself present for a friend who is sad, or you may find yourself becoming aware of a vigorous moment when you rise to a challenge. The contents of the moment are not as important as the feeling of being present. These are the moments when you feel present as you are. Not whom you think you should be. Again consider what you bring to those moments. These are your gifts. Write them down and try to describe them, giving them names like: generous presence, or still confidence or willingness to accept.

Play with this exercise for a couple of weeks. Don't take it too seriously.

Once you have discovered a few

You may want to use this sample notation in your healing journal to define your gifts.

August 25. Today I notice the pleasure I feel when warm water from shower slides down my back. I felt sensuously present. There was openness to the moment, like a pause. My body felt whole and awake. I noticed it later as I climb the stairs to put the laundry away and the later afternoon light poured through the window. The stairway suddenly became bathed in golden light. I stopped and felt the same openness to the moment. It was like a refreshing pause even though my arms were full of laundry. My body felt whole and awake. I call this gift, sensuous warmth of being.

of your gifts, image you are putting them on like a cloak. For example, in the morning you may think, today I will wear "gentle touch." The next day you decide to put on "laughing heartily at myself." At the end of the day, write a paragraph or two about what the day was like when you walk in awareness of your gifts. Become very familiar with the feeling tone of your gifts.

Then consider how your gifts are useful in the healing setting.
In this way you will become a confident and skillful healer who can

change and adapt, reflecting the needs of each healing.

Meditation

Peace Meditation

The peace meditation is one of the most important healing practices I know. It is with our senses that we experience the world we live in. Our senses are doorways. It is through our senses that we become aware of smiling faces, angry grimace, Bach piano concerto, and car horns. The smells of a garbage strike during the summer in the city or a rose garden both evoke memories and feelings in our hearts. These experiences, healthful and harmful, imprint themselves on our senses and obscure the clarity of our perception of life's many events. The peace meditation gently soothes any harmful memories that are embedded in your senses.

This meditation can be done lying down, sitting in a comfortable chair or in the traditional meditation posture of legs crossed while sitting on the floor.

To begin:

Make an aspiration toward peacefulness. (By the way, peacefulness is a very awake serenity.)

Bring your awareness to your breath. Breathe deeply into your belly. Be aware of the rise and fall of your belly.

When you feel grounded and let your breath find it nature rhythm and depth, quietly begin to say the word peace.

Bring your awareness into your right eye.

Imagine soft white light, the light of peace, entering your right eye and cleansing it.

It cleanses all illness and sights you have seen that have hurt you or you have turned from. These leave your eye in the form of soot, smoke, black tar and insects.

When you feel satisfied with the cleansing of your right eye, turn your awareness to your left eye.

Repeat the cleansing and continue to quietly repeat the word peace.

Now, when you feel satisfied with the cleansing of your left eye, bring your awareness to the space between your eyes.

Imagine white light entering and cleansing this area until you feel a balance between the two eyes. Continue to repeat the word peace.

Next turn your focus to your ears, nose and mouth. It is important to spend an equal amount of time on your right and left senses to create a sense of balance.

Bringing peace into your body

Starting at your feet, bring your awareness to your right foot, and cleanse it with the white light of peace.

Now bring peacefulness to your left foot.

Proceed up your body, alternating between the right and left sides.

At the third eye, become aware of your crown chakra, and bring peacefulness to this area, then:

Throat chakra

Heart chakra

Navel chakra

Root chakra

Location of Your Chakras

The crown chakra is right in the centre of your head.

The throat chakra is at the base of your neck in the centre.

The heart chakra is in the centre of your chest in front of the spine.

The navel chakra is three fingers below your navel just in front of your spine.

The root chakra is located just above your perineum.

Now move back up through your chakras checking the balance between the two sides of your body and from the crown, radiate peace to the world.

Radiating peace

Now, sit quietly radiating peace.

Share the peace.

Any the peacefulness I have gathered through this practice, I share with all others so they may be peaceful.   X3

Reflection

"Knowing that you love the earth changes you, activates you to defend and protect and celebrate. But when you feel that the earth loves you in return, that feeling transforms the relationship from a one-way street to a sacred bond."

Braiding Sweetgrass: Indigenous Wisdom, Scientific Knowledge, and the Teachings of Plants by Robin Wall Kimmerer

Understanding the Body/Mind

1. Over the next month, pay attention to taste. Try using the following questions to guide your awareness of taste. Make short notes on your observations.

❖ What tastes do you crave? Note time of day. What have you eaten during the day? What is your emotional state? What do you think this craving is about? Is something missing from your diet, life? Is the craving bringing you into balance?

❖ What tastes do you dislike? What are your associations with the taste?

❖ Which tastes do you mask? How do you mask them?

❖ Can you taste without judgment or association?

❖ Note how your body reacts to different tastes.

❖ Note how your mood responds to different tastes.

❖ Seek out foods or flavours you have not tried, note your process of exploring new tastes. Are you anxious or excited, or perhaps you experience other feelings?

❖ After trying a new taste: did you enjoy the taste, pretend you enjoy the taste or just spit it out?

❖ What is the relationship between taste and texture?

❖ Can you spit out what you do not like? Practice spitting out an unpleasant taste.

❖ Watch others and note their choices of tastes, their character and perhaps dominant element. Which element do they lack?

2. Pick up the following essential oils: lavender, rosemary and tea tree oil. Over a period of three days, have a bath using each oil. With lavender and tea tree oil use 10 drops. These can go straight into the bath. Add 10 drops of rosemary essential oil to a tablespoon of olive oil before adding it to the bath. Note the influence of each scent on your body/mind. Write down your observations.

3. Try listening to the following sounds and observe how the sounds affect your mind/body.

❖ Google Chopin's *Raindrop Prelude* and listen to it. Try to feel the music with your body. What do you notice?

❖ The wind on different days

❖ Water — rivers, fountains, taps, showers, rain, etc.

❖ Listen to the sound of 5 different people's speaking voices (tune out the words)

❖ Your heart beat (if you can't hear it try someone else's or your dogs or cats)

❖ Record your observations.

4. Ask someone to tell you about a problem they are having. As they tell you their problem, think about a solution to offer them when they finish speaking. How does this experience make you feel?

5. Ask another person to tell you about a problem they are having. This time you do not need a solution to their problem. Just listen. How does this experience make you feel?

6. Sit with a plant, a houseplant is fine, and ask it what it needs? Listen. What happens?

7. Sit in busy places and close your eyes, for example: a restaurant, shopping mall, office, etc. Record your observations.

Creative Monographs

Create a monograph in the form of a picture, song, story, or poem about the following plants:

Celery seed (Apium gravelons)

Slippery elm (*Ulmus fulva*),

Thyme (Thymus vulgaris)

Blackberry leaves (*Rubus fruticosus*)

Please see the monograph on Mint in the introduction to help guide you in the type of information you need to include in your creative monograph.

Enhancing Herbal Knowledge

1. Record the activity of the bitter taste on the body/mind. Name three bitter herbs.

2. Record the activity of pungent taste on the body/mind. Name three pungent herbs.

3. Record the activity of sour taste on the body/mind. Name three sour herbs.

4. Record the activity of the sweet taste on the mind/body. Name three sweet herbs.

5. Record the activity of the salty taste on the mind/body. Name three salty herbs.

6. Record the activity of astringency on the mind/body. Name three astringent herbs.

Medicine Making

Cold Medicine — An Infused Honey

In a jar, mix:

The chopped peel of one orange.

Slices of the orange that was just peeled.

Three cloves of garlic crushed.

1 piece of ginger the size of your thumb (grated).

2 tablespoons of dried thyme.

Cover the contents in liquid honey.

Put the lid on.

For the next two weeks, every two days have a teaspoon of the honey mixture.

Make notes on your experience.

What are the medicinal qualities of each ingredient?

Make An Apple Cider Vinegar

Pick a jar. (A large pickle jar, one with a wide mouth is a good choice.)

Gather the number of organic apples you would need to fill it up.

Cut up the apples into small pieces, saving the peels and cores.

Let the cut up apple sit exposed to air for a few hours.

When the apples are brown, put them in the jar and cover with spring water.

Cover jar with cheese cloth.

Stir the apples and water several times daily.

If the water evaporates, add more.

After a week of stirring begin tasting.

When it taste right, strain the apples and bottle the vinegar.

Medicine Questions

Why is apple cider good for digestion?

What advantage does it have for medicine making?

Dreams:

Try to notice your senses in your dreams. Many dreams are mostly visual with some sounds. See if you can taste the air of your dreams. Or smell the room you enter into during a dream. Can you feel the clothing you are wearing on your skin during a dream?

Over a period of a month, ask for a series of dreams to explore sensing. For the first three nights ask for a dream to enhance your understanding of sight. Then ask about hearing, smelling, taste and touch. Take a couple of nights off between each sense to let your dreams rest. Write down your dream even if it makes no sense.

How to ask for a dream

Before sleep, gently ask for a dream about a specific topic, problem, plant, body part. Anything you can dream up! Ask for the dream three nights in a row. The key is not to be pushy about the asking. Try to be humble and open when asking for a dream.

Catching your dream

Then catch the dream in the morning. To catch a dream, try to be very quiet when you first wake up. Alarm clocks are no friend to dreamers. Again gently ask yourself, what did I dream? One image or a textured feeling tone with an emotional quality may present itself to you. Accept whatever you are given.

Recording your dream

Before starting your day write down the dream in your dream journal. During the day, pull the dream back into your awareness and carefully reflect on it. After three days, look over the dreams you have recorded, like you are piecing together a puzzle or reciting a poem. Perhaps a sudden flash of intuition will flood your mind with a new understanding of the question you posed.

Lesson Three
The Physiology of Assimilation:
The Goodness of Life

Please read chapter three in The Herbal Apprentice: Plant Medicine and The Human Being.

Healer Heal Thyself

The Wheel of Time

As much as I wish I could transcend time, time affects my ability to absorb life.

What is your relationship to time? Is time a tool you use or are you a slave to time?

In this lesson you will have the opportunity to study your relationship with time.

In the life of an herbalist there are two different kinds of time. There is linear time. This is the time that our culture runs on. In linear time we arrive and leave according to the designated time told by clocks. We pay bills, have birthdays and celebrate holidays, create lists of tasks, exchange our time for money — all driven by linear time. As an herbalist living and practicing her medicine, part of my life is lived within the confines of linear time.

The other time a herbalist must respect is nature's time. It is late August as I write this. I am temporarily staying at a friend's home in Central Alberta. All around the house are wild roses. I have never seen rosehips so pump and bright red in all my years in Alberta. I really want to pick them to make winter medicine with before I leave here to return to a land where there are few wild roses.

I know the medicine in rosehips is not ready until after the first major killing frost. So I wait, wondering if the frost will come before I leave so I can take some hips with me. Or will I say good-bye to this place before the frost arrives and leave the hips for the deer and the rabbits? This is living by nature's time. Only nature knows when it's time plant, pick and make medicine. Although after a while one develops a sense of nature's rhythms, but let me make it clear rhythms are not schedules!

For example, in the spring, winds arrive. There will be a gusting wind that blows many branches off the poplar balsam trees. In the morning after the big wind, branches with buds oozing resin can easily be picked from the ground to make medicine with. Some people pick their poplar buds in the middle of winter. The resin (the medicine) is hard then and not such a sticky mess to work with. I, however, prefer to gather my buds from the ground, after the big wind, perhaps because the spring winds show me which buds to gather. Letting go of the branches in the big wind the poplar offers an herbalist medicine without needing to use her knife.

When my office was in a downtown environment, I always thought I was good at managing time during client meetings. I used to surprise myself how I could keep an appointment to two hours or one hour. Then I let go of the office and began seeing people in my home. My time management skills flew away! I had no ability to keep the appointment on track within a certain time limit. I could not understand what was so different. The information I took during the interview had not changed, nor did the physical exams. Then one day a client said to me, it sure is good not to have the parking meter ticking away down on the street when I come to see you! Then I knew, it was not some innate ability I had to keep an appointment on track, it was the awareness of parking meters and the penalty of a parking ticket that kept the appointments on time.

The challenge is one never knows when the big wind will blow. It might be on the day you have to meet with your bookkeeper to finalize your taxes. Or it might be during Easter when you have a house full of family and you are cooking a big dinner. Nature's time and linear time often conflict and this conflict is something the herbalist balances.

One more note about nature's time: healing takes place on nature's time. Birthing and death take place on healing time. Trying to fit any of these major life events into linear time complicates things quickly. Trying to make healing, birthing or death fit a schedule slows processes down. It's like picking medicine before the medicine is ready, you just should not do it. Why would you? (This is not a rhetorical question.)

I have a difficult relationship with linear time. I dislike the feeling of being pushed about by a clock and a schedule. Sometimes I think of linear time as the thief of joy. Too much time spent in linear time stresses me out! When I have time, I relax into timelessness and strangely feel I have more time.

People for a very long time have lived with nature's time, performing life-giving activities according to moon, day/night and seasonal cycles. It was only after we moved into cities and began to work in factories that time was broken into small measurable units like seconds and minutes. Time became something traded for money. Over time, we began to think of time as a "real" thing, a commodity. We use expressions like having time, spending time and wasting time.

Not all cultures have the same relationship with time. My Blackfeet friend, Tanya, gave me a teaching on Indian Time. I found this teaching very useful. "Indian time" can be a very derogative (perhaps racist) expression suggesting that First Nation peoples are irresponsible and lazy because of their lack of respect for linear time. But Tanya explained Indian Time like this to me, "It's about doing the thing that is most important in the moment." She went on to explain that when the willow is ready to pick in the spring, it is more important for her to do that then show up for the book club meeting. Or if an elder is dying, it is more important for the healer to be with the elder than to be at the conference he is schedule to speak at.

Indian Time is like Nature's time.

I have tried to live with doing what is most important in the moment. Of course this has challenged my priories — or what I thought were my priorities.

Once when I was having difficulty "managing" time, a friend told me about a Buddhist practice done to learn about time. He suggested every time I think about something, that I do it immediately. "Oh," I thought at the time, "that is impossible. I am always thinking about something to do!" But I tried it. Instead of thinking about returning phone calls, doing dishes, taking the dog for a walk, making an appointment to get my hair cut, getting the birthday card in the mail, talking to Mark about the ping in the car, etc. and etc., I did it! Strange as it sounds, I suddenly had a lot more time and was thinking a lot less.

Doing what is most important and foremost in your mind, changes your relationship with time.

As I said, I have a difficult relationship with time. When I have a difficult relationship, I take the advice of a Zen master — "Keep your enemy close."

It is always difficult to offer a definitive meaning for a Zen expression. This is my interpretation for "keep your enemy close."

When we don't like something, we try to get rid of it immediately! This often causes more problems. Just take a look at the garbage (in particular, plastic) crisis on this planet. Obviously throwing away garbage is not working. It is still in our midst causing much pain and suffering. Throwing away what you don't like is not "keeping your enemies close."

> Keeping your enemy is a useful expression to healers. It is important that you learn as much as you can about the person and the condition they struggle with before offering healing advice, if the advice is to be useful.

"Keeping your enemy close" means you learn everything about your enemy to gain an understanding of the interdependence of the difficult relationship. It is only with understanding that change can happen. For example, if we really understood the challenges of plastic in a meaningful way, we would probably return to carry things in baskets and clay pots. The same is true with our culture's difficult relationship with time.

So before you try to change how you live with time, learn *how* you live with time. Exploring these questions and exercises will help you understand your relationship with time.

Over the next month:

❖ Notice how you talk about time.

❖ How do you respond to time limitations?

❖ How do you feel when there are no limits on your time?

❖ Consider how your family and different family members use time and feel about time.

❖ Are you always early? Why?

❖ Are you frequently late? Why?

❖ Try being early or being late.

❖ Do you eat, sleep and have sex on time?

❖ How does being on hold on the telephone affect your awareness of time?

❖ What do you do while you wait?

❖ When do you first notice time in your day?

❖ Spend a couple of days moving slowly. Walk slower, drive slower, eat slower, shower slower, etc.

❖ Spend a couple of days moving quickly.

❖ How does movement affect your relationship with time?

❖ Stop every hour and notice what you are doing. Why are you spending your time in this way?

❖ How do you judge yourself for the way you use time?

(Why is time an important study for an herbal apprentice? Because successful herbalists have a great need for an exceptional relationship with both linear and nature's time.)

The Wheel of Time

Every healer I know would not disagree with a statement that goes something like this: Health is balanced.

Time is a great tool to measure how balanced your life is. Stress shrinks time. Relaxed states of mind expand time. How we spend time has a profound effect on how we carry our stress load or exhale into relaxation.

Let's explore how you use time to create balance in your life. Create a circle divide it into the following sections according to the amount of time you give to each part of your life on an average week.

The Wheel of Time will be different for each person, just as each stage of life will offer different ways we spend time. How a young mother spends her time, will look very different ten years later when she decides to return to school.

Health is being able to adjust to the needs of the moment. If in ten years when she returns to school, meeting her families physical and emotional needs continues to dominate her time, she will not succeed at school and it is quite possible her health will suffer from being driven by too many desires.

The Wheel of Time can bring to awareness the lacks in our lives, the parts of us that are not being nourished. How is time affecting your ability to absorb your life? The lack may be a temporary challenge. Other areas of life are demanding attention. This is okay for a certain period of time. However, if the lack becomes chronic, unhappiness and quite possibly health concerns will begin to push themselves into the Wheel of Time. Struggling with illness interrupts our relationship with linear time in the most disruptive way!

Spend some time creating Wheels of Time for your life. You can use the headings I have suggested or create your own. Perhaps you want to make a wheel with headings that are not so broad reaching. You may want headings with more precision such as time spent on Facebook, time cleaning the house, time hanging out with the kids, time with Mom, etc.

What does the Wheel of Time teach you?

Meditation

This meditation helps you learn the language of your body. It was developed from a very old meditation practice from the time of the Buddha called the 32 parts of the body.

I find this meditation helps me understand my body's needs, but at times I have found it helpful to understand my client's needs.

Many people find this practice quite challenging as it contradicts what many believe about their relationship (or lack of relationship) with their body. I recommend you take your time with this practice. Approach it with patience and curiosity, be persistent and your body will teach you more than any two-dimensional anatomy book.

Meditation on Your Guts

Breathe into your heart for a moment or two to center yourself.

Breathe into your liver. Explore your liver.

Ask yourself:

What texture is my liver?

What colour is my liver?

What shape is my liver?

From which ancestor did you receive my liver?

Does my liver have a feeling?

What does my liver need?

Image you are giving your liver what it needs.

Breathe into your stomach. Explore your stomach with the same questions.

Breathe into your small intestine. Explore your small intestine with the same questions.

Breathe into your pancreas. Explore your pancreas with the same questions.

After you have explored each organ, return to the sensation of your breath at your nostrils.

After a few breaths, share the practice with the following prayer.

Any understanding and compassion I may have gained about my body with this practice, I share with all others, may they have compassion for their bodies. 3xs

Reflection

Watch how you nourish yourself on fantasy, wanting, wondering, worrying, and on feelings of alienation. These constitute a bowl of worms.
A Guide to the IChing by Carol Anthony.

Understanding the Body/Mind

This winter I met a Mayan healer. It was during a turning point in my life. I was being challenged with letting go of an impossible dream and getting on with using the gifts I have or continuing to pour my energy into an unattainable dream at the expense of my gifts,. Needless to say, my digestive system was facing a number of challenges. In other words, caught at the cross roads, I could not digest my life.

The Mayan healer cornered me and through an interpreter strongly told me to listen to my guts before making any important decision. She emphatically stated, "I was ignoring the wisdom of my body." So I stopped and listened. My life changed. I am happier and my digestive system is better.

Let's practice understanding the relationship between your guts, your digestion and your life. Please try to see each question in this exercise as both an objective analysis of your digestive system as well as a metaphor on how you absorb your life.

❖ Once a day check in with your gut feelings. How would you describe your gut feelings? What is your relationship with your gut feelings? What triggers gut feelings?

❖ Pay attention to how and where you eat. How this effects your digestion?

❖ When chewing food, try to pay attention to the movement of your tongue? Are you aware while chewing or reading, talking or just thinking about something that has nothing to do with your meal?

❖ Exam your tongue in the mirror with a small flashlight. Is it red in colour, pink, lavender? Is it coated so that you cannot see the colour?

In very general terms:

  o A red tongue represents heat in the digestive system.

  o A pink tongue is considered a sign of health

  o A lavender tongue is a sign of a cold digestion.

  o A yellow coat is a sign of heat in the digestive tract.

  o A white coat is a sign of coldness in the digestive tract.

❖ Look at other people's tongues to compare the colour of their tongues to yours.

❖ If your tongue shows heat, try eating cooling foods for two weeks. Salad greens are cooling. You can also take cooling herbs, like demulcents, bitters and alfalfa.

❖ If your tongue shows coolness, try eating warming foods. Nourishing soups with ginger or a pinch of cayenne. Take warming teas like peppermint, rosemary or nettles.

❖ Notice any changes in your tongue colour and the health of your digestive tract. Write them down.

Creative monographs

Create a monograph, in the form of a picture, song, story, and poem, about the following plants:

Chamomile (Matricaria recutita)

Meadowsweet (Filipendulum ulmaria)

Fennel (Foeniculum vulgais)

Hops (Hummulus lupus)

Enhancing Herbal Knowledge

Differentiate between the following carminatives, which are energetically cooling, warming and heating.

Before doing any reading on these plants:

Drink three cups of peppermint tea for four consecutive days. Note your experience. Peppermint is a warming carminative.

Follow this by drinking three cups of lemon balm tea for four consecutive days. Note your experience. Lemon balm is a cooling carminative.

Drink three cups of freshly grated ginger tea for four consecutive days. Note your experience. Ginger is a heating carminative.

How do the energetics of the different plants interact with your body?

What do the books say the difference is between these three plants? Is this your experience?

Medicine Making

Garlic Oxymel created by Dr Christopher

8 oz. apple cider vinegar

¼ oz. caraway seeds (*Carum carvi*), crushed

¼ oz. fennel seeds (*Foeniculum vulgare*), crushed

1 ½ oz. garlic (*Allium sativum*), fresh pressed

10 oz. honey

Measure apple cider vinegar into glass pot, add caraway and fennel seeds. Bring to a boil and let simmer for 15 minutes. Remove from heat and add garlic. Let sit until cool. Press and strain the liquid. Add honey. Place onto low heat and melt the honey.

What are some of the medicine actions of caraway seeds, fennel and garlic?

Note some the medicinal effects of apple cider vinegar.

Note some of the medicinal effects of honey.

How would using honey or/and apple cider vinegar change the energetics of the herbs?

How might you use this oxymel?

Make Sauerkraut

If you are doing this lesson during any time other than harvest, you may have to wait to do this medicine making. Much medicine making happens when the timing is right, not when the herbalist is ready. By the way, this is one of the greatest challenges to being a medicine maker in this modern age.

To make sauerkraut:

Get yourself a large green cabbage that has just been plucked from the ground. It is important that the cabbage has not been sprayed with pesticides or wash with anti-bacterial soup.

Chop or slice the cabbage up. I prefer fine slices. Mark, my husband, prefers coarsely chopped cabbage. While chopping or slicing sing your favourite songs.

Stuff the cabbage in a large jar and sprinkle intermittently with sea salt.

With a large cabbage, you will need about 1/8 cup of sea salt.

Then press the cabbage down using your fists. (Still singing.)

Water should start to come from the cabbage and fill the jar.

Put an up-side-down plate (or saucer depending on the size of the jar) over the cabbage.

Put a jar or some kind of container full of water on the plate. The weight of the water in the jar should be enough to keep the cabbage submerged under the water.

Put a tea towel over the jar and wait a couple of days.

In a couple of days, lift the tea towel. If the water is evaporating add a little more and taste the cabbage. Cover again. Check every couple days.

After about two weeks, but everyone has a preference for how long they let their sauerkraut sit, put into sealed jars and pop in the fridge.

Eat two tablespoons daily and notice how your digestion changes. Of course keep notes. The notes will help during your next experiment with sauerkraut.

Dreams

For three nights ask for a dream about the health of one of your organs. Each night, write the question in your healing journal before you go to sleep. In the morning, write down your dreams.

Then for three nights ask for a dream about what the organ needs for greater wellness. Again write down the question in your healing journal. In the morning record your dreams.

Remember always ask for a dream with humble curiosity.

Sometimes when we receive a dream it is difficult to understand how it relates to the question we asked at night. Be patient it takes time to learn the language of dreams. If you are gently persistent one day you will recall a dream and have an Ah Ha! moment. In this moment the dream will suddenly fit together like pieces of a puzzle and you will understand one layer of its meaning.

One technique I use to understand dreams is to feel them in my body. To do this try sitting quietly for a moment, rest your mind on your breath, then when you feel ready recall an image from the dream. See if you can feel the image in your body. Or notice what feelings the dream image evokes. This will help you discover some of the non-verbal messages from the dream world.

Lesson Four
The Physiology of Circulation:
An Ocean Wrapped in Skin

Please read chapter four of the Herbal Apprentice: Plant Medicine and the Human Being.

Healer Heal Thyself

Heart's Desire

I am going to ramble a bit, like a wild crafter seeking a plant in an old growth forest. Forgive me.

The first steps into the forest.

The heart's desire is true to the Hippocratic oath — Do No Harm.

Following a well-traveled path

When I was in Herb School I had several part-time jobs in large public institutions. The pay was good and the schedules were flexible — these two aspects fit my student needs. However, like any other large institution built on the ideals of fairness and goodness, budgetary restrictions and legal considerations crept into the institution's good work like invasive weeds into the forest. Soon the institution's goodness becomes lost like indigenous medicine in clear-cut forests.

Budget restrictions and heaps of paperwork are formidable opponents of the goodness institutions aspire to. These limitations impede the heart's spontaneous joyful kindness. Personally, I was unhappy working in these institutions. My heart's desire for connection and caring were not welcome.

Unable to find satisfaction in my work, I took to shopping, looking for satisfaction in things and activities.

Resting. My back supported by an ancient Cedar, drinking water.

Then I graduated and I quit working for institutions. I opened The Green Clinic: Herbal and Traditional Healing and suddenly I stopped shopping. Even though the Green Clinic was just a small sapling, I found immense joy and satisfaction working with plants to help others. My heart's desire was being nourished. I no longer needed to shop.

This is not to say that the beginning of The Green Clinic was not difficult. Any sapling needs constant attention, the right soil to meet its needs, room to put down roots, sunlight for energy and frequent watering to grow. It did not matter that I had to work hard and had no money; I was happily following my heart.

When I began to practice plant medicine my connection to life on this beautiful planet grew like mycelium on the forest floor. Plant medicine's deep roots and its symbiotic relationship with human beings wove me into the wholeness of life in a way I did not know I was missing. Plant medicine anchored me in the interconnectedness of life on this planet. My heart's desire for connection was no longer sterilized by institutional rights and wrongs but became a fermentation in web of life. I was bubbling with nourishing joy. And like any fermentation, the abundance of life's giving goodness grew to beyond knowing.

Hopping on slippery stones across a stream

Recently I was personally (not professionally) entangled with a person suffering with border-line personality disorder. One of the primary symptoms of this mental illness is the difficulty experiencing empathy.

Empathy feeds my relationship with the rest of life on this planet. Empathy is the mycelium on the forest floor, the yeast on the wild apples bubbling into apple cider; it is the thread that binds me to life beyond my skin. I cannot fathom life without empathy.

Carefully I traced my interactions over the years with this person struggling with his inner emptiness: the emptiness of empathy. As I think back I become confused in the maze of his stories that included accounts of debits and credits, what is owed and what is paid. His legal arguments and statistics numb my mind. His relationship to life on this planet is a contract fixed with words that are rigid with meaning. There is no room in his life for dancing beyond the boundaries of right and wrong, mine and yours, and entitlements.

Empathy is a leap beyond the black and the white; the red of blood, the green of chlorophyll, the turquoise of lakes fed by glaciers and dark grey skies bringing storms. Empathy is like Earth accepting everything, receiving everything, nourishing all of life without discrimination.

Listening to bird song

Empathy opens me to life. It helps me suspend belief and move beyond knowing. It allows me to forgive. Empathy pushes me to a deeper understanding of my connection with every breathing life form birthed by our planet. I simply cannot imagine living without empathy. A life without empathy must be painfully lonely and unbearable at times.

I have asked many people to meditate on their heart's desire. Most people, using their own language, tell me their heart's desire is to connect with others, to be deeply involved with life, to discover a visceral knowing of belonging. Many tell me their heart's desire is to give back to life in a meaningful way, to be present with life, to respect life. If I had to put my heart's desire into words I would say it is allowing the pull of empathy's thread to weave me fully into life.

Sinking in soggy moss

We have all at times been infused with loneliness and the threads that connect us to life become tangled in low self-worth and self-hatred's sharp thorns. Luckily for most of us, something happens: a child is born, someone dies, a ray of sun falls across the living room floor, a cat purrs on your lap... life knocks us out of our loneliness and we renew our connection to breathing, dancing, laughing and grieving life on this planet.

Coming upon a meadow where roses bloom.

I strongly believe empathy will not allow harm! It is my experience that empathy is the great healer. Empathy, like water, quenches the thirst of every living being on this planet. Empathy offers the healer the chance to transcend gratitude and learn to give back to life in the most meaningful way. Plants give those who use them with respect the medicine of empathy.

Finding the medicine, making offerings and getting dirty digging up roots

In this lesson explore your connection to life and your heart's empathy.

What do I mean when I say pay attention to the quality of your mind? This can be a confusing exercise for some people. To begin to identify the quality of your mind, think of your mind like water. When you consider the quality of it, what form is the water taking?
Is your mind like fog?
Or is it more like a very still, crystal clear lake?
Perhaps it feels like a muddy puddle?
Angry minds are like a pot of boiling water.
Comforted minds may seem to be like a jeweled drop of dew cradled in the velvet softness of a ladv's mantel leaf.

In your Healing Journal

Make notes on the following:

1. Go for a walk. Step gently on the earth. Open your ears to the sounds around you. Sniff the air. Touch plants as you pass by. As you walk, think or say to yourself, "Belonging."

2. Study connections. Notice when you feel connected to others. Scan your body; learn the physical sensations of being connected to life. Notice how connection affects the quality of your mind and the feelings in your heart.

Discovering Physical Sensations
Some people have difficulty describing physical sensations that are not overtly painful or pleasurable. If this is your challenge, begin with describing physical sensations as being either hard or soft. In mediation practice, hard and soft sensations are represented by the earth element. They are generally the easiest to discover. Then move on to discover inner feelings of warmth and coldness. This is awareness of the fire element.

---

3. Notice when you have lost the thread of connection. Scan your body. What are the physical sensations of isolation? Notice the quality of your mind when you lose connection and feelings in your heart.

4. In your Healing Journal write about moments when you have felt most connected to life. Study those moments. How did they come about? Who was there? What were you doing? Is there something similar about each moment or is each moment different?

5. Actively initiate awareness of your connection to life every day. You may do this with a prayer, a ritual, a smile at a stranger or a welcoming caress on a plant's leaf. Discover your ways of connecting.

6. If you were a plant, what kind of plant would you be? You can draw it, make a monograph of it, and write a poem, perhaps a dance, any way to describe yourself as a plant. It might be a real plant or a mythological plant. How does being this plant fill your heart's desire? How does this plant connect you with life? Play.

Meditation: A Heart of Gold

Gold is the colour of the earth element in its purest form. Gold is a colour of strength with flexibility. Gold represents richness. This meditation will help you develop a strong connection with your heart, giving your life both flexibility and richness.

To begin:

Settle into your body and rest your mind on your breath. You may wish to use turtle meditation to ground yourself.

Once settled:

Imagine a gold light about an arm's length above your head. It is warm, calm and vibrant. Sense it, feel it, open to the gold light above your head.

Imagine a gold light about an arm's length below your feet. It is warm, calm and vibrant. Sense it, feel it, open to the gold light.

Imagine a gold light about an arm's length in front. It is warm, calm and vibrant. Sense it, feel it, open to the gold light.

Imagine a gold light about an arm's length behind. Lean back into the light. Feel how it supports you. It is warm, calm and vibrant. Sense it, feel it, open to the gold light.

Imagine a gold light about an arm's length to your right. It is warm, calm and vibrant. Sense it, feel it, open to the gold light.

Imagine a gold light about an arm's length to your left. It is warm, calm and vibrant. Sense it, feel it, open to the gold light.

Imagine a gold light in the four quarters. It is warm, calm and vibrant. Sense it, feel it, open to the gold light.

All the lights join up and you are sitting in an egg of gold light.

Rest for a moment. Explore how you feel in the gold light, your body and your mind.

Now, gently begin to breathe into your heart center, just in front of the spine, behind the sternum. As you breathe into your heart, a sparkling gold star appears. Let your breath explore the star.

As you breathe in and out of the star in your heart, you notice the star's light shines and connects with the golden egg surrounding you.

With each breath, gold light swirls from the star touching the surface of the egg and swirling back into your heart.

Enjoy breathing with light for as long as you want.

Now...the golden egg dissolves into your body.

Your body dissolves from your feet and your head into the star in your heart.

On the next breath, the star dissolves.

Rest, quietly for a moment.

Share the peacefulness of the practice with others.

Reflection

Teach love, for that is what you are. – George Elliot

A Study of the Elements

Water: Circulation of Rivers

Explore rivers. Find a map of North America and follow the flow for major rivers, like the North Saskatchewan, the Colorado and the Mississippi from their sources to their final union with the ocean. Trace their tributaries. Examine how the watershed of these rivers change as the river widens. Explore the history of rivers and their relationships with human beings.

If you live near a river, visit it regularly. Discover how it changes with the season. How does its colour change? What affects the way it flows?

Notice the wellness of the plants on its banks and the animals that come to it to quench thirst.

Learn about estuaries.

Study other bodies of water: puddles, sloughs, lakes and even clouds and fog.

Understanding Body/Mind

Discovering your circulatory system

- ❖ Draw a diagram about how the heart receives blood, pumps it into the lungs, receives blood from the lungs and pumps it into the body.
- ❖ What is the difference between arteries and veins?
- ❖ Take time each day to listen to your heartbeat. If you have a drum, play the heart beat rhythm. Listen to heart before and after you have played your drum.
- ❖ Put your hand over other's hearts and feel their rhythms. I like to feel my dog and cat's hearts beating.

Listening to the Pulse

This is a fire/air element exploration.

Spend an evening in candlelight only. How does it affect your mood? Feel your pulse at the end of the evening. Describe it.

> **How to find the Pulse**? You can easily check your **pulse** on the inside of your wrist, below your thumb. Gently place 2 fingers of your other hand on this artery. Do not use your thumb. This is called the radial pulse. You may have to press deeply or lightly touch the wrist depending on the character of the pulse.

Spend an evening on the computer. How does it affect your mood? Feel your pulse at the end of the evening. Describe it.

Feel three other people's pulses, both the right and left. What do you notice? Record your observations.

Creative monographs

Rosemary (*Rosmarius off.*)

Hawthorn (*Crataegus oxyacantha*)

Linden flower (*Tilia Europa*)

Cleavers (*Galium aparine*)

Cayenne (*Capsicum annuum*)

Prickly Ash (*Zanthoxylum americanum)*

Enhancing Herbal Knowledge

How would the following classes of herbs affect circulation? (Studying the chart on Herbal Actions in lesson 3 may help you.)

1. Circulatory stimulants
2. Diuretics
3. Alternatives
4. Diaphoretics

Medicine Making

Castor Oil Poultice

Make a castor oil pack and place it over your liver three consecutive days in a row for 20 minutes. Note any effects the pack has on your body.

Four days later, repeat the process and make notes on the process.

How to: Soak a large flannel cloth in castor oil. Place the cloth over your liver and cover with a hot water bottle. This is very relaxing. Leave the poultice on for 20 minutes.

Do this for three evenings, rest for four evenings, and repeat 2 to 3 times. You can reuse the cloth several times. Wrap it in a plastic bag after use to preserve its medicine. Castor oil can be purchased at drug stores.

Note: You may wish to place a plastic bag over the castor poultice to avoid staining the cloth on your water bottle or wheat bag.

How does using a castor oil pack effect your circulation?

How would adding 5 drops of ginger essential oil to the poultice effect the action of it?

Rosemary Hydrosol

You need:

Large saucepan with a lid.

Old fashion metal vegetable steamer with holes in it. Remove the pole from the middle.

Small bowl.

Bag of ice.

Distilled water.

Find four to five bundles of fresh rosemary at the grocery store.

Directions (

1. Chop the rosemary and place in a large saucepan.
2. Cover the rosemary with water to about the width of a thumb nail.
3. Place the vegetable steamer into the water on top of the rosemary.
4. Place the bowl in the middle of the vegetable steamer.
5. Put the lid on the pot, upside down.
6. Bring the water and rosemary to a simmer.
7. When steaming, place the bag of ice on top of the lid.
8. Wait a bit.
9. Take the pot off the heat. Let cool.
10. Take the lid off and collect the water in the bowl. This is your hydrosol.
11. If you think there are more oils left in the rosemary, repeat the process.

How would you use the hydrosol?

Dreams

Like any good storyteller, dreams evoke an atmosphere that supports the unfolding of its story and the symbols. One of the most effective ways to understand the language of your dreams is to explore its atmosphere.

There are many, many ways to describe the atmosphere of a dream. The atmosphere may describe the dominant emotional state of the dream such as excitement or perhaps confusion. Or it perhaps the dream is cloaked in an ancient or otherworldly atmosphere.

The easiest way to do this is to ask yourself, "What was the atmosphere of the dream?" Sometimes I find this question enough to discover the underlying importance of a story line or set of symbols that appear quite random or mundane on the surface.

To deeply explore a dream's atmosphere, I settle into a quiet inner place and bring to mind a specific symbol or part of the dream. Then I ask myself, "What is the feeling of this dream symbol?" If my mind is quiet enough, my body will respond to the symbol and question with a particular sensation that suggests an emotional energy pattern. I know this may sound strange to you, but try it. Your experience will be your teacher.

One of my favourite ways of playing with a dream is to choose a symbol that seems to be of no particular significance, such as when I dreamt I was pouring water into a teapot. When I recalled the symbol of the kettle and asked, "What is the feeling of the kettle?" and waited for my body to respond, I discovered layers of meanings to the dream I never could have imagined if I had only used thought processes.

Try this technique with a dream that baffles you and see what happens.

Here are the steps:

1. Quiet your mind/body.
2. Bring to mind the dream or a specific dream symbol.
3. Ask, "What is the feeling of the dream or symbol?"
4. Let your body respond.
5. Make notes in your journal.

Lesson Five
The Physiology of Defense:
It's All About Healthy Boundaries

Please read chapter five of *The Herbal Apprentice: Plant Medicine and The Human Being.*

Healer Heal Thyself

Protection and security are BIG themes in our world.

An important question every healer needs to ask herself sometime or another is: How do I protect myself?

Many healers take out insurance policies and wrap themselves in white light. Locked doors, child-proof caps and credentials are another form of protection healers seek. Unfortunately, although these things decrease risk, they do not guarantee security.

In the loving-kindness meditation we pray, "May happiness be my guard." This prayer suggests that happiness is a form of protection. It has certainly been my experience that loving-kindness and happiness is a form of protection. When my heart is open to others, insults and injury roll off my back. A slower reaction time solves many problems.

Quick reactions, not rooted in loving-kindness, generally create entrenched positions, hurt feelings and blaming attitudes. Quick reactions are rarely solution orientated and lead to more fear about living our joy, offering our gifts freely and expressing the truth of our being creatively.

Realistically though, it is almost impossible to sustain a continued state of loving-kindness. At times we all react quickly, dig a trench, nurture our wounds and blame others. Beyond the idealism of a continuous state of loving-kindness, we are left with the question, "What is protection?" or "How do I protect myself?" Knowing how unpredictable life is, I'm stumped for an answer.

When a question does not bring forward a creative solution to a problem, I reframe the question. Let's try the question this way, "As a herbalist, what am I protecting myself from?" One answer that resonates loudly is — mistakes!

Oh the dreaded mistake! We all fear them. Images of fingers pointing at you saying, "It's your fault!" "You're to blame!" "How can you call yourself an herbalist when this happens!" Mistakes are looming shadows in the dark corners of most healers' minds. Perhaps fear of mistakes is a form of conscientiousness because as herbalists we know mistakes lead to discomforts for our client like constipation or diarrhea, skin rashes, a sleepless night or worse — scary anaphylactic reactions.

We know, if we have studied plant medicine and human beings well enough, that there is always a chance that something unpredictable can happen with our medicine, as with any medicine. With a mistake, will we be blamed, sued, reviled? With this thought a blank arises in the mind quickly filled with images of ridicule and disgrace.

What if there is another reason to make mistakes? What if mistakes can be a form of protection? Now that is radical! Is fear of mistakes a form of protection?

I know it's a cliché but I am going to use it anyways, *We learn from our mistakes.* (Using clichés are mistakes writers make!) By carefully retracing the steps we made along the path to the mistake we will learn how not to make the same mistake twice. Discovering the underlying causes of a mistake, whether it be an oversight on your part, a challenge with the plant medicine itself, or something not disclosed by the client, you will learn how to ask better questions, how to source and examine your plants whether fresh or dried, and how to keep yourself aware and present.

I used to think if I was right, I could not make a mistake. Then if I did not make a mistake I would be safe. Therefore, I invested time and energy into being right. Fortunately, I made mistakes. Eventually, a realization broke into my hard headedness (part of the cause of some of my mistakes) and I learned being right is not a form of protection. It only causes more mistakes.

Being right means one cannot listen to other points of view. Hearing other points of view often offers the important information needed to avoid mistakes.

I have found mistakes such a remarkable opportunity to understand practical (and often not recorded) information about plant medicine. Mistakes have taught me to gently probe my clients until I have received all the information I need to make good recommendations on the use of plant medicine. Mistakes have made me a better herbalist. Honestly and openly acknowledging my mistakes offers me the protection of integrity.

When I have made a mistake in my practice as a herbalist the first thing I do is acknowledge it and talk about it with the client. I clearly express my sincere regret and offer free replacement medicine or their money back. Interestingly, rarely does the client want free medicine or their money back. Usually they are relieved to talk about the mistake with me. They value the opportunity to clarify the cause of their experience. Most (and there has not been a lot of mistakes in my practice) clients who had unfortunate experiences using plants I offered are my most loyal supporters. They know they can trust me to be honest with them and that I am willing to listen to their concerns. This is the best protection I know.

As an herbalist you will make mistakes. You might as well accept this now. And you might as well prepare yourself to be open and honest about your mistakes. If you are smart, you will vow to learn from them the first time and not the second, third, fourth and so on.

Most people learn to protect themselves from mistakes by either blaming another person or venomous self-criticism. These are strange forms of protection. In my experience both of these reactions to mistakes only creates more harm. Openly acknowledging mistakes creates a sense of vulnerability. In vulnerability, there are no shields between ourselves and others. Vulnerability is just two humans looking at each other allowing all to be seen. Nothing hidden. Allowing yourself to be vulnerable is the great healing. Your mistakes will take you there. We are always vulnerable no matter how much we shield ourselves.

So let's begin to shift our attitude towards mistakes. In your healing journal explore the following questions.

    1.   Write about a mistake you made that you covered up.

Why did you not acknowledge the mistake?

How did the mistake make you feel at the time?

What did you learn from the mistake?

How do you feel about the mistake now?

2. Write about a mistake you openly acknowledged.

How was the open acknowledgement of the mistake received by others?

What did you learn from the mistake?

How do you feel about the mistake now?

3. Write a commitment to yourself about how you will respond to future mistakes. Honour your commitment.

Meditation

Meditation on Giving and Taking

The meditation practice in this chapter is an adaption from a Tibetan practice called Tonglen. In my life I have found this meditation very useful as a means to become peaceful with conflict and to find solutions to problems that are outside of my usual ways of thinking.

Giving and taking meditation is traditionally practiced to develop a compassionate heart. It is the compassionate heart that is fearless and is open simultaneously to many different viewpoints. Having a compassionate heart is essential for the healer. A compassion heart is profound protection.

I have taught this meditation practice for many years. Often people recoil at the basic premise of this practice — taking on another's suffering. So let's spend a bit of time exploring what it means to take on another's suffering before trying out the practice.

Get ready for a radical statement! It is natural for human beings to want to take on another's suffering. Or putting it another way, a compassionate heart is the basis of the human being. Or, try this one on — it is unhealthy to feel alone, isolated and not connected to the rest of life. It is healthy to have an open, compassionate heart.

When most people hear of a friend's loss, heartache is felt. When we see images of mass suffering caused by an earthquake or war, our hearts ache. When we hear stories of children being abandon or abused, our hearts ache. When we feel a loved one's pain, our hearts ache. This heartache we collectively experience is compassion.

The compassion we feel inspires actions. We send a card or make a call. We give money to ease financial hardship. We raise our voices against injustice. We cook food for another. We donate blood. We listen, hold hands, send a prayer. Compassionate action has many forms.

The important piece to remember is the ache we feel in our hearts arouses compassionate action. The practice of giving and taking helps us become comfortable with the ache of compassion so we do not turn away, become overwhelmed or simply complain and let someone else do the heavy lifting.

It is also important to understand about this meditation that it is a teaching of transformation. A compassionate heart does not hold onto another's suffering. It transforms the suffering — like making lemonade out of lemons. The practice of giving and taking is not about swallowing another's pain and letting it rot out your guts. This practice is about having confidence in the power of your own goodness and compassion to transform another's pain.

Begin the meditation:

- ❖ Clearly state your aspiration.
- ❖ Bring your mind's focus to the nostrils and count ten breaths.
- ❖ Recollect moments of kindness in your day.
- ❖ Turn the kindness into a beautiful, peaceful white light in your heart.
- ❖ Breathe into and out of the light.
- ❖ Bring to mind a challenge you have that you would like to offer healing to.
- ❖ Imagine the challenge in front of you.
- ❖ Breathe in the suffering caused by the challenge in the form of smoke.
- ❖ Let it mix with the white light of your heart.
- ❖ The smoke transforms in the white light and the light becomes brighter.
- ❖ From your heart, breathe the light into the heart of the challenge in front of you and continue to offer healing.
- ❖ Continue until you feel satisfied.
- ❖ Return to your breath at the nostrils and count 10 breaths.
- ❖ Return to the sphere of gold light.

In an attitude of prayer say, "The goodness that has come of this practice I share with all." Imagine gold light spreading.

Reflection

You don't protect your heart by pretending you don't have one. –
Anonymous

A Study of the Elements

In a fire pit, a fireplace, or a wood stove build a fire. Before you build
the fire, practice turtle medicine meditation and center yourself with
your breath. Try to catch the very moment when the flame moves from
the match to the paper. Study how the flame moves across the paper
and begins to lick the wood. Listen to its sounds. Feel the heat spread. If
you are doing this at night, notice have the fire light shines into the
darkness. Quietly watch the fire for some time. Feel how your
body/mind responds to the fire. What do you notice?

Understanding Body/Mind

The immune system is all about relationships and boundaries. The
health of your immune system reflects your relationship to your body.
The following exercise, called Writing Your Body's Story, will help you
understand the complex weavings of your relationship to your body and
perhaps the early roots of the dynamic exchange between you and your
skin, flesh, bones and blood.

We all have a personal story about our relationship with our body. Our
body story includes discovering fingers and toes, pleasure and pain, the
colour of skin, eyes, hair. Our body story involves how we create
movement, the experience of hunger, peer pressure, trips to doctors,
our mother's and father's ideas, etc.

The story of your body has plots and subplots. Many experiences shape
our relationship to the body: sex, birthing, nursing and having friends
become sick and die. We may personally experience illness that
profoundly influences our body's story. As each event, conversation and
belief is woven into our flesh and mind, our story of our body becomes
a personal mythology.

Write the mythology of your body. Try to pay attention to events that
shaped your belief about your body and influence your relationship to
it. Try to spend time with story, make it more than a page long. Avoid
writing a body story that sounds like a list of symptoms, clinical test and
diagnoses you may offer to a doctor or herbalist. Write a story about

feelings, sensing, intuitions and understandings about your body. Write about your identity and your body.

After writing the story, read it to a good friend and talk about any insights that arose from the writing and reading of the story.

Leave the story for a couple weeks and then return to it. Read it and then make notes about further insights and patterns you recognize.

Dragon Tracks

There is a saying in Traditional Chinese Medicine that, "The dragon leaves its tracks on the skin." The dragon in this case means illness and disease. Study the skin of different people, even just the skin on their face. What do you see? How does the skin change with health, acute illness and chronic illness? How is the immune system involved in these changes?

For more about skin and its dragon tracts check out these two books:

Reading the Body: Ohashi's Book of Oriental Diagnosis

by Wataru Ohashi and Tom Monte

Field Guide to Clinical Dermatology (Field Guide Series)

by David H. Frankel

Creative monographs

The herbs you are studying in this chapter all have pronounced effects on the immune system. As a herbalist it is very important for you to be able to differentiate between plants that stimulate the immune system from those that moderate the immune system. While studying the plants below please keep this in mind.

It will also be useful to you to consider how and when you would use these plants during chronic or acute illness. Ask yourself, "are these plants slow to respond or is their medicine fast acting?" Please also pay attention to dosing of these plants. Finally, research traditional ways of offering the medicine of these plants. For example: astragulus is offered in a bone broth soup while chaga is prepared with several decoctions; find out how echinacea was used to treat snake bite.

If you learn these plants well, you will have a strong understanding of how to support the immune system with plant medicine.

Astragulus	*(Astragulus membraneous)*
Chaga	*(Inonotus obliquus)*
Rhodiola	*(Rhodiola rosea)*

Echinacea   *(Echinacea agustifolia)*
Elecampane   *(Inula helenium)*

Enhancing Herbal Knowledge

1. What do the herbs in the creative monographs have in common?
    How are they different?

2. Determine if the following actions are organ specific, affect a
    physiological function or help return the body to balance
    (physiological imbalance). You may want to refer to the Herbal List
    of Actions in appendix 1.

    Thyme   *(Thymus vulgaris)*
    Red Clover   *(Trifolium repens)*
    Goldenseal   *(Hydrastis canadensis)*
    Marshmallow *(Althea officinalis)*
    Plantain   *(Plantago spp.)*

    How would each of these plants affect the physiology of defense?

3. Note the primary effects of adaptogens on the body. How do these
    herbs affect the adrenal glands? Can you differentiate between the
    used of Korean ginseng (Panax ginseng), American ginseng (Panax
    quinquefolius) and Siberian ginseng (Eleuthrococcus senticosus)?

4. The following herbs are classed as anti-inflammatories. How each
    herb would affect the inflammatory process in the body.

    Nettles (Urtica dioica)

    Meadowsweet (Filipendulum ulmaria)

    Turmeric (Curcuma longa)

    Marshmallow (Althea officinalis)

    Cleavers (Galium aparine)

Medicine Making

Steam Inhalation

Try a steam inhalation using these two different techniques.

Method one:

1. Boil a kettle of water.

2. While waiting for the kettle to boil collect the following:
   - a large bowl
   - a ¼ cup of dried thyme or sage
   - a large towel or blanket.
3. Put the dried herbs in the bowl.
4. When the kettle boils, pour the water over the herbs in the bowl.
5. Put your head over the bowl and cover yourself and the bowl with the towel or blanket.
6. Breathe deeply.

Method two:

Replace the dried herbs with 5 – 10 drops of essential oil of thyme or sage and repeat method one.

Makes notes on your experience. Which method do you prefer and why? Which would you use for a child of 5 years of age?

Bone Broth

In a large pot combine:

   A whole chicken cut up

1 onion

3 cloves of garlic

1 tablespoon of astragulus root to each cup of water

1 tablespoon of apple cider vinegar

Cover chicken with water

Simmer at a low temperature of 4 to 5 hours, adding more water is needed.

Strain.

Pick chicken off bones and add back into the broth.

Freeze in ½ cup portions.

Take one portion per day. You can add vegetables if you wish when warming the soup.

Do some research on bone broth. How does bone broth support the immune system? Would you use a bone broth with astragulus during an acute or chronic condition?

Medicinal Wine

For each of the following dried herbs:

Rosemary (Rosmarinus officinalis)

Sage   (Salvia officinalis)

Cinnamon (Cinnamomum spp.)

Choose a favoured wine. Red or White. You may also choose sherry or port.

1.   Pour 500 mls of your chosen wine into a jar.

2.   Grind up 100 grams of your chosen herb in a coffee grinder.

3.   Add the herb to the wine.

4.   Put the lid on tightly and shake.

5.   Label the jar with the date, herb and wine. In a separate place record the amount of herb used and the amount of wine.

6.   Put the jar in a cupboard.

7.   Shake daily for two weeks.

At the end of two weeks, strain the wine, and press the herb with cheese cloth.

Re-bottle and label.

Try it out.

Dose: 1 tablespoon 2 to 3 times a day in a ½ cup of water.

Make notes on your experience of the medicine-making process and the effects of the medicinal wine.

How can you improve on this recipe?

Dreams

The ancient Greeks had a deep appreciation for healing dreams. Before Hippocrates and his appreciation for humoral medicine, the Greeks turned to the god Asklepios for healing. (Hippocrates was initially trained in this tradition. I suspect that dream healing did not suit his dominant thinking function!)

For healing, ancient Greeks travelled to temples dedicated to Asklepios to consult with a physician/priest. The physician/priest would recommend a series of cleansing rituals that included fasting, healing baths and massage.

Each person seeking healing would also attend theatre performances that re-enacted the many tragedies of life (hence the Greek Tragedies).

These plays depicted the death of loved ones, infidelity, betrayal, abuse, war, disease, loss of status, etc. The physician/priest used the tragedies as a form of psychotherapy. It was the hope that the tragedies opened up the profound insight that personal pain is reflecting suffering common to all of life. This understanding eases ego identification with personal misfortunes and opens the heart to compassion for the suffering in all of life. This is similar to the medicine of the meditation giving and taking.

After the baths, the good food, the herbal medicine, massage and psychotherapy, the supplicant was sent into the dream chambers deep within Asklepios' temple to seek a healing dream.

It was believed that Asklepios, the healing god, appeared to offer advice on healing or brought the patient back to health solely through dream. There were three primary symbols that represented Asklepios: an old man, snakes and dogs. If a dream included one of these symbols, it was taken very seriously.

Over the next few weeks ask your dreams for healing symbols. Record the symbols you dream of each night.

Pick three symbols that either re-occur or carry a potency for you and create a list of associations for each symbol. (Potency may be reflected in a discomfort with a symbol or in a strong attraction to a symbol.)

For example: In the dream I am walking along a path dark forest and I almost step on a snake.

Snake: Kundalini energy, healing, cold blooded, evil, poison, forked tongue, knowledge, shedding skin, transformation.

Dark forest: Hard to see, wild animals, trees, where the witch in fairy tales lives, easy to hide, hard to find medicinal plants, earthy smells, green, sound of wind in trees.

Path: Where one walks, the path of awakening, dirt, tree roots, not well travelled, but others have travelled before me.

Interpretation: Because I almost step on the snake that represents healing and knowledge, as well as life force, while in a dark forest on a narrow path, one interpretation would be that parts of myself that have been unconscious are being brought to consciousness, although they still cannot be seen in "the light of day." The path I am travelling on during this healing journey is known to only a few. I must practice constant awareness not to miss healing opportunities, as they are difficult to see. Loss of awareness (stepping on the snake) may result in a loss of life energy.

For more information on Asklepios read: *The Practice of Dream Healing: Bringing Ancient Greek Mysteries into Modern Medicine* by Edward Tick, PhD.

Lesson Six
The Physiology of Letting Go

Please read chapter six of *The Herbal Apprentice: Plant Medicine and the Human Being.*

Healer Heal Thyself

Living in an Ideal World

The Dream

Several years ago on New Year's eve I had the following dream:

I am in a large parking arcade. It has several floors like the type attached to a large mall. It has many, many cars parked in it. I am wandering through the cars looking for mine. I am carrying my agenda/date book for the following year when a strong wind blows through the parking arcade causing my agenda to fly from my arms. The agenda/date book is blown open and all the papers where my plans are recorded are scattered about the parked cars. At first I run about trying to gather up the swirling papers. Then I stop and realize I will never be able to gather them together again.

Before this dream, on New Year's Day, I'd write down my goals for the following year and include plans to attain them. Since that dream, I have not set a single goal on New Year's Day. (Or on any other day for that matter.) At first I felt almost naked going into a New Year without a vision of what I wanted to achieve in the coming year. It seemed counter intuitive to success — getting what I wanted.

After the dream, and without goals, it was not long before I realized I felt more content with my life. It seemed without goals I was able to flow more easefully through each day. The following New Year's Day I reviewed how a lack of goals had affected my life. I realized it had been one of the more fulfilling years in my life and I had accomplished a great deal more than when I set goals. It was my first year; I paid taxes on the extra earnings I had made as a herbalist.

I realized that a plan about how my life should move forward limited my ability to respond to opportunities as they presented themselves. Without a plan I was able to see opportunities that otherwise I might have ignored as they did not fit into my agenda. Without a set plan, I was able to respond each moment as it arose instead of trying to create the content for each moment. The dream helped me see that I needed to get out of success' way. My agenda needed to be eliminated for me to succeed.

The Circle

A number of years ago I was sitting in a circle with a group of young healers. We were sharing our future dreams. Three women envisioned having a beautiful healing centre. They spoke about the places they dreamt of creating for people and animals to come for healing. They described the types of gardens they would have, what the buildings looked like and how people would be nourished, cared for and healed. Their dreams were inspiring but something felt unreal about them.

Within a couple of months, one of the women became pregnant. Her and her partner bought a house and she decided to devote herself to her newly forming family. About six months after the circle the second woman came to the conclusion that she did not like being around sick people and took up painting. She told me had never felt happier. The third woman kept her dream of a healing centre alive.

Daily she wrote about it. She painted it. She told people about it. Unfortunately, the more energy she put into dreaming about her healing centre the unhappier she became. She grew to dislike her home where she had her clinic. "It's not big enough," she complained.

She fought with her husband, "He just does not get the big picture," she whined. She believed he was hindering the realization of her dream. She even found her clients exasperating, "They just don't work hard enough at their own healing." She felt they were not the type of people who would be attracted to a healing centre.

The more she wrote about her healing centre, the more she hated her life. Nothing she did in her "real" life compared to the beauty of her dream. Nothing she did measured up to her ideas. She needed a BIG wind to blow away her agenda.

My teacher Cecilie often reminded me that, "Ideals are the cruelest task masters."

Before we delve deep into elimination let's explore ideals.

Why are we looking at ideals within the context of elimination?

Ideals tend to be very, very pure. Snowy white actually. Ideals are clean, lacking mishaps and life's many toxins. Elimination processes tend to get rid of the used up, dirty toxins of life. Before we explore elimination and toxins, we need to understand what we believe to be pure — our ideals.

In your healing journal explore the following:

1. Write a page about your ideal life.
2. Write a page about your everyday life as it is currently manifesting.
3. Compare the two pages. See if you can sense a difference in the feeling tone of each description.
4. When you were a child of about 5, what did you want more than anything?
5. Consider the above question again when you were 10, 15, 20, 30, 40 and so on. How have these longings been met? How important are they to you now?
6. Describe a moment in your life when your ideals came down to earth. How did this moment change you as a person?
7. What ideal are you willing to let go of today?

Meditation

Breathing Rainbows

This meditation cleanses the energy body and opens up new possibilities. It is a fun, joyful meditation practice. This meditation is adapted from a tradition called the Seven Rays of Healing.

To begin:

Face the sun. You can be standing or sitting outside (or sitting in a sunny spot inside).

Image the spectrum of light from the sun coming into your body.

Breathe deeply in the colour violet and feel it move through your body.

Then breathe the violet colour out, imagine it carries away any toxins or unhappiness in a sooty grey shade to the violet.

Repeat with:

Red

Orange

Yellow

Green

Blue

Do each colour three times.

Let the meditation change each time you do it. Let the rainbow breathe you.

Remember: do this facing the sun but not looking directly at the sun.

Try to do this practice for every day two weeks. Notice how the colours change. Notice the colours you are drawn to and the colours you have difficulty inhaling.

Reflection

Remember that sometimes not getting what you want is a wonderful stroke of luck. – His Holiness the Dalai Lama

A Study of the Elements

Consider how the elements engage in processes of revitalization. For example: Study the plants that grow in disturbed soil. How do plants rejuvenate the soil?

Look for dirty water. What processes clean the water?

Notice the difference in the air between a city and a forest. How is air cleaned?

How does fire participate in renewing an environment?

How can you mimic these processes to increase your well-being?

Understanding Body/Mind

What goes in must come out, is a fundamental law of good health. My very old dog hobbles about. But for a very old dog, she is in good health. How do I know? She eats and poops, drinks and pees, and breathes in and out.

An herbalist is always very interested in what goes into the body/mind, and in what form it comes out. The patterns of elimination will help you discern whether to use stimulating or relaxing herbs. Or perhaps you will not even need to use herbs, maybe you will just need to recommend more water or vegetables.

1. Pay attention to relationship between your bowel movements, food choices, stress, timing and water intake. Notice the frequency, colour, texture and smell. Make a chart and note changes over a period of a month. (See if you can talk someone else into making a chart and noting changes as well.) Compare the two charts, constitution and overall sense of well-being.

2. Pay attention to your urine. Notice its relationship to food, water intake, timing and stress. Notice its colour, smell, frequency and amounts as well as the particles in it. Make a chart and note changes over a period of a month. (See if you can talk someone else into making a chart and noting changes as well.) Compare the two charts, constitution and overall sense of well-being.

3. Pay attention to how emotions change your breathing.

4. Explore three ways you can cleanse every day. Try doing these three things for a week. What do you notice?

Creative monographs

Every system, organ and cell in the body is involved in the elimination process. Many cleansing regimes focus primarily on the bowel and kidney. The liver is also burdened with the sole task of elimination of toxins in many people's belief system. A cursory study on plant medicine however demonstrates that nature offers humans many ways to remove wastes from the body/mind. The following herbs help the body remove wastes. Each herb has a specific system it supports. When creating your monographs, keep in mind the whole body and how the particular system the herb focuses on supports the whole body.

Milk thistle   (*Silybum marianum*)

Dandelion   (*Taraxacum officinalis*)

Mullein   (*Verbascum thapsus*)

Red Clover   (*Trifolium pretense*)

Corn silk   (*Zea mays*)

Burdock   (*Articum lappa*)

Chamomile   (Matricaria chamomilla)

Enhancing Herbal Knowledge

1. What are the different effects of relaxing and stimulating herbs when encouraging eliminating processes in the body?

2. List two herbs from each class: stimulating expectorants, laxatives, and diuretics.

3. What are the signs that a condition requires stimulation to aid elimination when offering herbs for the lungs, bowel and kidney?

4. List two herbs from each class: relaxing expectorants, laxatives and diuretics.

5. What are the signs that a condition requires relaxation to aid elimination when offering herbs for the lungs, bowel and kidney?

Medicine Making

Create a cleansing smoothie

While creating a smoothie, keep in mind all the different ways to cleanse the body/mind. For examples, green vegetables are both cleansing and deeply nourishing, lemons are used to cleanse the liver, apples support elimination from the bowel. Make notes on how the plants you use in your smoothie are both cleansing and nourishing.

Create a Mud Mask

Clay is dirt. There is a certain appeal to using dirt for cleansing. So let's get to the dirt of cleansing.

Clay is a drawing agent. It cleans pores deeply. It helps to draw out excess oil from our skin and is an excellent therapy for those suffering with acne. Clay will also draw out poisons. It has long been used as a remedy for poison ivy, poison oak and even insect bites.

Whatever is applied to the skin is absorb into our body. Having been mined directly from Earth, clay is full of minerals that nourish the skin and body. When using clay, your body is absorbing the goodness of the earth.

Different types of clay to use for drawing toxins from the body:

Bentonite clay: This clay is very mild and suitable for most skin types. It gently draws toxins from the skin. This clay can be encapsulated and taken internally. Be sure to drink lots of water if you choose to do this. I also caution you to only do this for a short period of time as this clay has a powerful drawing effect of nutrients as well as toxins.

Pink clay: The pink colour of this clay comes from its iron content. It is specific to oily skin because of it powerful drawing properties. Pink clay, made into a paste and smeared over the liver has a deeply cleansing action.

Other ingredients in the mask:

Honey: moisturizes and cleanses skin.

Lavender: smells wonderful and strongly anti-bacterial

Making the mask

1/2 tsp of clay

Slowly add warm water until pasty consistency and mix thoroughly add:

¼ tsp of ground lavender flowers, grind in coffee grinder

¼ tsp of honey

Other ingredients you may want to try are: yogurt; add essential oils; try different herbs like comfrey or calendula or even mash up an avocado and add it.

Gentle Laxatives

Often in clinic, herbalists offer individuals support with laxatives. But for different reasons herbs containing anthroquiones, the bowel stimulating constituent in many herbal laxatives, cannot be used. For example: anthroquiones can cause contractions in the uterus for women in their 1st trimester.

Try making this stewed fruit recipes and have it on a cereal or porridge in the morning. Notice its effect on the bowel. What other benefits do stewed fruit have?

Granny's Stewed Fruit

1/2 cup prunes, cut them into quarters

1/2 cup Thompson raisons

1 cup pitted figs, cut in half

1 cup dried apricots, cut in half

3 apples, core and cut into pieces (leave the skin on)

2 pears, core and cut into pieces (leave the skin on)

Mix together in a pot. Add enough water so the bottom of the pot is covered and there is about an inch of water. Bring to a gentle simmer, put the lid on and simmer until apples are soft. If too thick, stir in more water.

Note: For minerals: add 1 tsp. of molasses.

Store in the fridge.

Dreams

Many dreams dislike being interpreted with words. They dislike having a "meaning" put on them. Many dreams are a reflection of feelings. Some feelings cannot be expressed with words. Sometimes words are like the lid on a pot that contains fragrant steam. The lid does not allow the steam to infuse the kitchen with its scent. Words can stop feelings from infusing a dream.

Word interpretation of dreams are often associated the left side of the brain. Feelings are more associated with the right side of brain. To access the right side of the brain's interpretation of the dream, draw the dream with your non-dominate hand. Because few of us use our non-dominate hand to perform tasks requiring fine motor skills, it is difficult to draw the symbols of the dream down in a neat and tidy manner. The dream symbols, when drawn with the non-dominant hand, become messy, unruly and difficult to manage, much like feelings. Drawing the dream this way will open you to the deeper feelings the dream is mirroring to you. The interpretation may not be made with words from your brain, but your guts will understand its meaning in the most visceral way.

Lesson Seven
The Physiology of Regulation:
The Nervous System & The Order of the Soul

Please read chapter seven of *The Herbal Apprentice: Plant Medicine and The Human Being.*

Healer Heal Thyself

Resisting Your Soul's Desire

Webster's definition of resistance: the refusal to accept or comply with something; the attempt to prevent something by action or argument.

A psychologist's definition of resistance: is the phenomenon often encountered in clinical practice in which patients either directly or indirectly oppose changing their behavior or refuse to discuss, remember, or think about presumably clinically relevant experiences.

In clinical practice a herbalist needs to support a client in taking their medicine. It is not unusual to hear a client say they were too busy to make their tea, or they never made it to the grocery store to pick up the avocadoes, or they kept forgetting to take their tincture or they left their medicine in their desk drawer at work so they couldn't take an evening dose.

There are many, many reasons for people to not take their medicine. Sometimes the medicine is too bitter. In that case I recommend taking it with some honey. Sometimes the client dislikes the taste of peppermint and I substitute another plant. If the client finds the protocol too complex, I simplify it. Sometimes, no matter how the herbalist supports the client, she continues to find reasons not to take enough medicine to effect change. In this situation the herbalist and the client are both facing resistance. Resistance is much trickier to work with than recommending honey to offset a bitter taste.

The only way to help a client overcome resistance is to learn about resistance in your own being. Follow these steps to discover resistance in yourself.

1. Identify one thing you have done in the past that was both interesting and supported your well-being. Remember when you stopped doing this activity. This activity might have been meditating 10 minutes during the day, writing down dreams in the morning, going for a walk or sipping an evening tea.

2. Now ask yourself why you stopped doing this activity. What was the reason you told yourself about ending the activity?

3. Give yourself a quiet moment, centre in yourself using your breathe and then tell yourself the reason you stopped the activity. If the reason you no longer write down your dreams, or meditate, or walk is true you will feel yourself sink into your body. If it is not true, you will experience a flurry of mental activity that shores up the story you have told yourself. If this is the case, you have discovered resistance!

Sometimes I think resistance is like coming up against a glass wall. You can't see it, but you can feel it.

The important thing about resistance is — it is an initial sign that healing is moving deeper into your body/mind. Resistance is like the guardian to the cave of inner knowing. Resistance asks you, "What or will you give up in order to receive? What price are you willing to pay for being whole, healthy, creative, joyful, etc.?" It is the moment when you ask yourself, "Am I willing to surrender to this change?"

The challenge with healing is we never really know what change it will bring to our lives. It is impossible to know exactly what we will find in the cave of inner knowing. We can easily use expressions like wholeness, authenticity, love, healing, connection and other vague warm and fuzzy terms to express what we believe or hope to find in the cave of inner knowing. But if one does not know these ways of being while standing on the threshold of change, the discomfort of change (also called resistance) can cause one to turn away from entering the cave and choosing the path of distraction.

Standing on the threshold of a deeper healing we are asked to surrender our current truth for something unknown. This is uncomfortable. The greater the change is, the greater the discomfort becomes. In order to avoid the discomfort we stop meditating, writing down dreams, journaling, taking our flower essence, or whatever it is that is helping to bring in the new way of being and get busy. Somehow we believe, "If I stop doing what is causing the discomfort everything will be okay."

The path of busyness or Netflix binging or a box of donuts or a new love affair or shopping works for a while, maybe a day, a week, a month, maybe even a year. The further down the path of distraction we wander the more the threshold of the cave of inner knowing becomes misted over. Then suddenly one morning one wakes up feeling stuck and knowing something has to give. Probably what needed to be surrendered to enter the cave of inner knowing.

Struggling in stuckness, one seeks another healing modality or return to the one left behind. The process starts all over again until resistance is met. Standing on the threshold of change, one more time you are asked to embrace the discomfort of resistance, surrender or leave behind the healing. It is up to you.

Inquiring into Your Soul's Desire: Overcoming Resistance

This is a journaling exercise in which you answer three questions. As you answer these questions in your journal let yourself write without a censor and try not to take your pen off the page. See if you can write two full pages for each question, notice when resistance arises and just keep writing, even if it's just, "I don't know what to write."

You may want to allow a week between journaling each question. This exercise does not need to be done in an hour. But if you want to, it can be.

Question 1: Who are you?

Question 2: What happens through you?

Question 3: What's missing?

Question 4: What is your soul's desire?

Question 5: How does your spirit support your soul?

(This exercise is an adaptation of "Who are you?" from Joanna Macy's book Coming Back to Life.)

Meditation

Meditation on equanimity

Equanimity is a kind of mental balance that is not disturbed by outer events in life. It is said the Buddha was moved by either pleasure or pain. He knew each had arisen due to specific to conditions and would pass when those conditions were no longer present. This understanding creates equanimity. Equanimity is never leaving the cave of your heart to chase outer satisfaction or run from outer dissatisfaction.

Another way of looking at equanimity is that it is being in a place where you are always ready to let go. Of what are you letting go? Mostly points of view. Perhaps you should just do the meditation and you will see what I mean.

To begin...

Settle and centre yourself.

Image you are standing on a path. It can be any kind of path in any kind place. Most importantly you are standing on a path.

Facing you is someone who is your friend.

Image you take a step back. The step represents 2 days ago.

Still facing your friend, think, "What was I doing 2 days ago, what was my friend doing?"

Take another step back. This step represents 2 weeks ago.

Still facing your friend, think, "What was I doing 2 weeks ago, what was my friend doing?"

Take another step back. This step represents 2 months ago.

Still facing your friend, think, "What was I doing 2 months ago, what was my friend doing?"

Take another step back. This step represents 6 months ago.

Still facing your friend, think, "What was I doing 6 months ago, what was my friend doing?"

Take another step back. This step represents 1 year ago.

Still facing your friend, (although your friend is slowly moving away from you) think, "What was I doing I year ago, what was my friend doing?"

Take another step back. This step represents 2 years ago.

Still facing your friend, (your friend continues to move away from you) think, "What was I doing 2 years ago, what was my friend doing?"

Take another step back. This step represents 5 years ago.

Still facing your friend, (your friend continues to move away from you) think, "What was I doing 5 years ago, what was my friend doing?"

Take another step back. This step represents 10 years ago.

Still facing your friend, (your friend continues to move away from you) think, "What was I doing 10 years ago, what was my friend doing?"

And continue moving back in time by 5-year increments until one of you is in the womb. Then finally, do the exercise before either of your conceptions. For example: You are younger than your friend. Image where you were before conception, and where your friend was at that time.

After doing this with a friend. Try it with a family member, enemy, neighbour, etc.

This is a good meditation to make notes on. I often find unusual bits of information about my journey with this person come into view. This practice can also be useful to discover past life connections if that sort of thing interests you.

Do you understand how this meditation helps one let go and just be with what is?

Reflection

If I were a carpenter, I would build you a window to my soul. But I would leave that window shut and locked, so that every time you tried to look through it all you would see is your own reflection. You would see that my soul is a reflection of you."
— Colleen Hoover, *Point of Retreat*

A Study of the Elements

An elderly farmer once said to me in the last week of March when the winds were blowing from all directions bringing all sorts of weather that, "The north and south wind were battling over the land." Years ago I lived in a meditation house called: The Winds of Change. The Tibetans tell stories of a mythical horse called the Wind Horse who travels swiftly through the air carrying prayers of peace around the globe.

Study the wind. How does it bring change?

Understanding Body/Mind

1. Become aware of the relationship between your digestive system and your nervous system. Describe what you notice. For example: how hunger affects your nervous system or how digestion affects your sleep, how eating certain foods affects your nervous system, etc.

Create a chart to help you develop an understanding of neurotransmitters and plant medicine. Use the following headers:

Neurotransmitter	Action in the mind/body	Yin or Yang?	Signs of imbalance	Balancing Plants
GABA				
Serotonin				
Dopamine				
Norepinedrine				

Creative monographs

The following plants are all nervines. I would really like you to pay attention to the energetics of these plants and keep in the stimulating and relaxing effects in terms of energetics. Also, try to define these herbs as either tonics or effectors. Again refer to the chart in chapter 3 for more on effectors and tonics.

One thing I find particularly interesting about nervines is their relationship with systems other than the nervous system. See if you can find information about how these plants interact with the whole body/mind complex. For example: St. John's Wort was originally considered a hepatic.

St John's Wort (Hypericum perforatum)

Wild Oat Seed (Avena sativa)

Scullcap (Scutellaria laterifora)

California poppy (Eschscholzia californica)

Valarian (Valerianna officinalis)

Motherwort (Leonurus cardiac)

Enhancing Herbal Knowledge

How do the following plant constituents interact with the nervous system?

Volatile oils   (hint: look at peppermint and lavender)

Saponins (hint: look at Licorice)

Flavonoids   (hint: look at gingko)

How do bitters affect the nervous system? Name three bitter herbs routinely used to support the nervous system.

Medicine Making

Poplar Infused Oil

This is your second wild crafting exercise. Generally this medicine is made in the spring sometime around mid-April.

Go out and identify a stand of poplar balsam trees (*Populus balsamifera*). Be careful not to choose a stand of trembling aspen (*Populus tremuloides*). As I have written before, I generally wait until the spring winds have blown a number of branches off the poplar and gather my buds from those on the ground. If you cannot find branches on the ground where leaves are about to begin to unfurl, gather buds off a number of trees. Don't forget to ask permission from the tree and give it an offering.

Collect buds to fill a jar. (I generally use a 500 ml canning jar.)

Remove the stems and place the buds in the jar.

(Don't forget to sing)

Cover the buds with grape seed oil.

Place the jar in a croc-pot and surround the jar with water.

Gently heat for 12 hours.

Strain, bottle and label.

>How will you use the oil? Have a bath and add a ¼ cup of the oil to the bath. How does this affect your nervous system?

Healing Baths

Baths are an underused but important part of herbal medicine. Water is naturally calming for most people. Add a few herbs and you can calm and sooth the nerves, pain, infections and skin conditions. For example: chamomile baths for colicky babies, oat baths for dry itchy eczema, lavender baths for insomnia, chaparral baths for yeast infections, rosemary baths for revitalizing, and many more.

I have two challenges with herbal baths:

1. I find you need a lot of herbs to make them effective. Because of this I often sip herb tea while in the bath. (Sort of lazy, I know.)

2. Loose herbs in the bath make a big mess to clean up. This not pleasant particularly after a very relaxing bath. I make a cheese cloth sack to contain the herbs. (Some people make bags with panty hose, but I find panty hose as one of the most annoying remnants of the patriarchal culture and refuse to have them in my house or office.) Or make a very strong tea and add it to the bath water. It depends on the herbs.

Try these two baths:

Oat Bath

2 cups of regular oat flakes (not quick oats)

Grind them to powder. A fine powder.

Sprinkle the oat powder into the bathtub as it is filling with water. You may have to stir it up a bit.

Get in and enjoy.

Calendula Path

1 cup of dried or fresh flowers in a large teapot or cooking pot.

Bring 4 cups of water to a boil.

Pour the water over the flowers and cover.

Let steep for an hour.

Strain and pour tea directly into the tub.

Light a candle, turn off the lights and get in.

Make notes on both baths. Why would you recommend each bath?

Dreams

If you have been writing down your dreams, you will have quite a collection of them by now. Read through the last few months and look for reoccurring symbols. Make a list that includes the symbol and the date.

For example: different forms of transportation often occur in dreams:

Dream October 17 - Black bicycle, my mother driving.

Dream October 30 - Black car, I am in the back seat and do not know who is driving.

Dream November 1 - Red convertible whizzing by.

Dream November 10 – Black car, red interior, my husband driving, I am in the passenger seat

Dream November 30 – Pink Cadillac, like a Barbie doll's, sitting on a shelf

Dream December 10 – Black motorcycle in garage

Dream December 15 – Old pick-up truck -A man shows me how to fix a flat tire on a country road

Dream December 22 – In a Volkswagen bug - driving by myself through winter mountain road, very slippery.

Dream January 3 – Buying a new green car.

Can you see how the symbol changes and shift

Lesson Eight –
The Physiology of Reproduction: The Vessel

Please read chapter 8 in *The Herbal Apprentice: Plant Medicine and the Human Being.*

Healer Heal Thyself

The Healing Thought

A friend of mine once wrote a poem about a calf dreaming itself into being while in its mother's womb. I once read how geese sleep during their long migratory flights. The writer imagined geese dreaming as they flew overhead in long v-formations. What do they dream I wondered? Do they dream one dream as they cross the autumn sky?

The thought of these unusual dreamers sparks a change in how I relate to the world around me. Baby calves and wild geese dreaming their journeys offered me a greater sense of wonder for this fragile yet incredibly durable, miraculous and hopelessly flawed world we all inhabit. The wonder of dreams in wombs and flying geese. Wonder opens me up and I ponder: what can I not know?

Questions like this lift us beyond the mundane realities of our lives — the cleaning, filling the car with gas, sorting socks, paying bills — you know all those things that take up our days until we have so little time to notice the miracles of being and we forget!

A woman's body is a wonder. It can incubate life. No one knows exactly how conception occurs. We know an egg and sperm come together.

DNA mingle and life is created. But life, to me at least, appears to be something beyond measurement. It is too big and elusive for a microscope. It's chemistry too complex for a centrifuge. Its meaning too ungraspable for labels. I may not know what it is that comes together to create life, but I am sure it is more than an egg and sperm coming together.

We cannot name precisely the intelligence in cells that forms the curve of the nose, or creates toes that hug each other tightly, or determines the unique swirl of a fingerprint.

I know women who have dreamt the name of the child they carry before seeing her face. Her name was April the voice said in the dream. Who named this little girl?

The life giving wonder of a woman's body is a mystery.

To all you beautiful men out there;

I apologize for not writing about the male body. I apologize for only exploring female reproduction. I promise in the future I will write about the male body, its challenges and the ways we can support healthy male balance.

I feel the core issue I write about, a mechanical view of the body, also traumatizes boys and men. I also believe that adolescence for males is a difficult time. Very little information about the changes that occur as a boy becomes a man is rarely spoken about with clarity, tenderness or understanding. Mostly though, it is my understanding that sexual trauma for boys and men — many believe it frequently occurs as sexual abuse toward women — is rarely spoken about, even more rarely understood and healed.

Please read what I have written about women's bodies and consider your own male body. Think about how your body is seen by others, how you see your body and explore deeply your experiences and beliefs around sexuality and reproduction as a male.

My heart aches for all the beautiful women who have been deeply traumatized in both their sexuality and birthing.

Without questions that ask how a woman dreams of unborn child's name, we begin to create a mechanistic view of the body, the uterus, life. Seeing the body as a machine makes it easy to treat it as one, something mechanical, without feeling, without sensing, without an intelligence of its own. We treat women's bodies like machines with convenient birthing methods, pills to dull its pain and to regulate its timeless cycles. Birthing and sex become distorted by a lack of feeling. Dignity is lost.

We inflict trauma, from birth to death, on our bodies as we believe, like a machine we should be able to control the discomfort of difficult emotions, not feel physical pain and experience pleasure with every whim. After all most of us live in a push button world, where we get what we want with the simple touch of our finger to a number. Why should we not have the same control over our bodies?

After trauma, and repeated trauma, bodies become numb and lose the power to feel. They become like a machine. A numb body lacks creative thoughts, dreaming descends into darkness and translucent grey veils distort our perceptions of the world, removing the wonders of life. Life's miracle vanishes in a litany of petty complaints. Our life becomes as repetitive as an assembly line.

By ripping away the veils and caressing the feeling back into the body, disrespectful views of our bodies fall away. Whether your body is juicy and plump or strong and athletic, or long and elegant, women need to learn how to cultivate kindness, dignity and respect for their bodies. This is not easy to do. Although we make more money now (and seem to have a lot more responsibility) and can vote in many countries, are allowed to divorce, and have choice of our sexual partners, women continue to be seen as a sexual commodity everywhere.

Sometimes I wonder if it will ever be possible that all women's bodies be given the dignity they deserve while sex sells. But because calves dream their way into being, I believe anything is possible. Life is wonderful. Let's discover the dignity of your body.

In your healing journal:

To discover where you carry dignity in your body, explore the following questions and ideas in your journal.

- Write about a time when your genitals where treated disrespectfully.
- Give your vagina a voice. Write what your vagina would say to the person or event that created the feeling of disrespect.
- Write about your first period.
- Write the advice you would like to give to the following woman:

- o An adolescence girl who has just begun her period.
    - o A woman who about to go on the pill in order to avoid pregnancy.
    - o A woman about to give birth for the first time.
    - o A woman who has just had a miscarriage.
    - o A woman who has just had a hysterectomy.
- Your body/mind is a miracle. Write about what you find completely fascinating about your body/mind.

Meditation

The Peaceful Goddess in Your Root Chakra

Begin by creating a forest green globe around you: Image green lights about an arm's length from your body in all ten directions. Then join the lights up to create a globe.

Rest in the globe for a moment.

Place your awareness at the top of the green globe and express your aspiration.

Breathe into your belly for a moment or two.

Breathe into your root chakra (which is between your genitals and anus) and notice it is the source of the green light.

Continue to breathe into your root chakra for a little while and slowly feel the green light from your root chakra expand.

Feel the green light fill your body, and the globe.

Rest for a moment.

Imagine there is a vibrating sound in your root chakra, a humming sound.

Begin to quietly make the humming sound.

Sense, feel the vibration of the sound, listen to the hum sound.

Become aware that the sound deepens the colour green.

Rest for a moment.

Now the hum turns into a serene Goddess.

Breathe in and out of your root chakra, allowing your breath to touch the Goddess.

Notice that the Goddess is breathing.

Consider the qualities of the Goddess. (Is she peaceful, energized, generous, determined, etc.?)

Imagine with each breathe the Goddess is breathing these qualities in and out, throughout your body, filling the green globe.

Rest for a moment.

Let go of the boundaries the globe creates around you and feel the green light now fills all of space.

Rest for a moment while the Goddess continues to breathe into your being and the world around you.

Notice that the Goddess breath becomes a fine golden thread

The golden thread weaves a web, connecting your breath with the breath of every living being.

Rest for a moment.

Now dissolve the practice.

Imagine the golden thread dissolves into the Goddess.

Imagine the green light dissolves into your body.

Your body dissolves into the Goddess.

The Goddess begins to dissolve, feet and head, until only the vibrating sound remains.

The sound dissolves.

Rest for a moment.

Share the merit: May any peace I have gathered with this short meditation practice be shared with all others so they may be peaceful.

Reflection

If I were a carpenter, I would build you a window to my soul. But I would leave that window shut and locked, so that every time you tried to look through it all you would see is your own reflection. You would see that my soul is a reflection of you.
— Colleen Hoover, Point of Retreat

A Study of the Elements

Study how the earth element changes into the spring with its interaction with the other elements. Notice at what point the earth becomes capable to bring forth seeds. What is the balance of elements that makes new life possible? How can you relate this to the environment of the uterus?

Understanding Body/Mind

Set up a system that a woman could use for increasing her awareness of her cycle. What do you think are the important events during the cycle that would you recommend she take note of?

Name five effects estrogen has on the body/mind

Name five effects progesterone has on the body/mind

Name five effects testosterone has on the body/mind

Name five effect cortisol has on the body/mind

Creative Plant Monographs

Raspberry leaf (Rubus ideaus folia)

Chaste-berry (Vitex agnus-castus)

Licorice (Glyccrihiza glabra)

Vervain (Verbena hastate)

Blue Cohosh (Caulophyllum thatroid?)

Sheppard's purse (*Capsella bursa*)

Yarrow (Achellia millifolium)

Enhancing Herbal Knowledge

Why would you want to include adaptogen herbs in a formula to support a woman with PMS or during menopause?

Why is dandelion root (Taraxacum officinalis radix) often added to a formula to support hormonal balance for a woman?

Differentiate between black cohash (Cimmicifuga racemosa), blue cohosh (*Caulophyllum thalictroides*), chaste berry (Vitex agnus-castus) and vervain (Verbena officinalis).

Medicine Making

Tea to support Breast Feeding

Choose five herbs to create a tea to support a breast-feeding mom. Keep in mind the taste of the herb (no one will drink a bitter tea several times a day), the availability of the herbs, the purpose of the herbs and the solubility of the plant's medicine. You need to decide how much of each herb will go in the formula.

Experience is the greatest teacher when formulating a tea and understanding the amount of each herb to use. So be prepared to make a few mistakes. Remember though to keep good notes and learn from your mistakes.

I learned to create formulas by dividing the formula into different amounts up to 100 grams. Many herbalists use the parts system. For example:

Totalling formula to 100 grams	Using parts for measurement
15 grams – raspberry leaf	1 ½ parts – raspberry leaf
20 grams – nettles	2 parts – nettle
20 grams – lemon balm	2 parts – lemon balm
35 grams – fennel	3 ½ parts - fennel
Total 100 grams	

Choose one way to create the tea and make your tea. Taste your tea and share it with a couple of friends. Do they enjoy the tea? Find it nourishing? If not, try again.

One more tip. Different parts of plants have different weights and take up different amounts of space in a tea blend. Here are a few pointers on using different parts of plants.

1. Flowers – light weight and can take up a lot of space in a tea.
2. Seeds – tend to be heavy and will make their way to the bottom of the bag.
3. Leaves – vary in weight and volume ratios.
4. Roots – tend to be heavier and often need longer time in the tea pot or thermos than other parts of plants in a tea blend. They may even need to be decocted.

Creating a Glycerite

Glycerites are made with glycerine and water. Sometimes a little brandy or vodka is added to a glycerite to help preserve the medicine. It has however been my experience that glycerites have a decent shelf life, so I only add alcohol if I need it as part of the extraction process.

To begin this assignment:

1. Research glycerine. There are two kinds. Which kind do you use in medicine making?
2. Why would you choose to make a glycerite as opposed to a tincture? I can think of three good reasons. I am sure there are more.

Make a dill glycerite

In a 500 ml jar add:

100 grams of dried dill – not powdered

Mix in a separate container

220 mls of glycerine

100 mls of distilled water.

Add the liquids to the herbs in the jar.

Put on a lid. Label. Make notes in your medicine making book.

Put in a cupboard and shake daily for 2 weeks.

Strain. (Any ideas why water was added?)

Taste. Put in a brown bottle, label and make notes.

Why would you offer this medicine to a breast-feeding woman?

How would you offer it to a child?

Dreams

For the next month record your dreams on paper with no lines. Write one dream on each page. Before recording a dream, draw a circle on the page and write your dream within the circle. Use only nouns to record your dreams in the circle.

For example: Instead of: I was walking down the road when I big bird landed on my head. In its beak was a worm. I took a hat out of my purse and put it on in case the bird dropped the worm on my head.

Road bird head beak worm hat purse bird worm head.

After writing the dream in the circle using only nouns, see if you can feel each symbol in the dream with your body.

Consider the comments that are beneath the video. What do you think is going on with the different results and effects?

Lesson Nine:
The Physiology of Movement

There is no corresponding chapter in *The Herbal Apprentice: Plant Medicine and The Human Being*. Stay tuned for the 2nd edition.

Healer Heal Thyself

Letting the Question Move You

This April morning, I checked the buckets hanging from the old sugar maples. They have been growing down the lane for 100 years or more. Some people call them Wolf trees. When they were planted they were the only trees in the clearing. This allowed them to stretch wide into the sky. The diameter of their trunks is a two-person hug: one person on each side of the tree, reaching until her hands clasp the person reaching from the other side of the trunk. Because they had room to reach for the sky without the hindrance of other trees growing around them, they are called wolf trees.

The maple's sap begins to flow in this part of the country after the first thunder-storm. Although the sap is running now, I did not hear a thunderstorm. Perhaps I was sleeping deeply that night and the thunder was distant.

The earliest sap is mostly water. I like to think of the first waters being pulled into the tree as flushing out the tree's clogged arteries, opening up its circulation after a long winter of hibernation. The first waters wake the tree. In a spring cleanse, a nettle tea will do this for the body — clear away the winter sludge.

As the ground thaws and the maples awaken, the water, pulled deep from within the ground, trickles through the woody roots, gathers stored sugars and begins its journey to the high branches touching the sky.

Over the next couple of weeks, the sap becomes sweeter and richer in minerals. The sugars in the sap nourish both the trees and maple syrup lovers.

The key to good maple syrup is waiting for the nourishing sweetness to arise and not be satisfied with the initial offerings of early spring.

Healing is a lot like sap rising.

To heal one begins with a question, though the question may not be clearly articulated initially. It might first be felt as a discomfort. One might muse: Is there something more? Or do I have to feel this way? Or perhaps I do not have to love like this? Is there another way?

The initial question is like spring thunder. It can be a roaring storm, raging across the sky for all to hear. Or it may be a quiet rumble in the distance, barely noticed while you dream of other things in the night. Be assured: to wake up the sap of healing somewhere a question is asked that challenges the way things are, both inside and outside.

The initial moments of healing open up pipes clogged with repetitive thought patterns and emotional responses. Some people are content to rest here at this phase of healing. They recognize a thought pattern and replace it with one that they feel suits them better. The pipes become unclogged in this way and new ways of being begin to wake up.

For the next phase of healing, to drink deeply of the sweet nectar that flows from the very roots of life, one needs to be willing to ask the harder questions. The questions we avoid. Or in other words the answers we take for granted. The hard questions shake us awake to the fragility of our personal life. By asking hard questions we are nourished by the sweet nectars that remind us we are a thread in the web of life.

Just as the maple tree needs to be patient, wait for the ground to thaw in the warm spring sun before being revived by the minerals of the earth and last year's sugars, in healing we must be patient and not settle for the simple answers. We must wait for the hard questions to arise that break through the deeper layers of our being and open us to the love of inter-being.

Try this:

Often we think of meditation as a something we do that has no movement. However, I have often found that it is movement during meditation that allows questions to penetrate deeply into my being, bringing forth the nectar of compassion and wisdom.

Go for a walk. A long walk, but not too long. By yourself. Take your time and look around. Ask yourself, "What is going on?" Ask yourself this question many times during the walk. What happens? Write down your observations in your healing journal.

Go for another walk. Much like the last one, only in a different place. Try to choose a place where there are other humans. As you walk and look around say to yourself, "I approve." Several times. Write down your observations in your healing journal.

Go for one final walk. Again similar to the walks you have already taken but in another location. As you walk, touch the things you pass and ask, "What is this?"

Write down your observations in your healing journal.

Think about how the questions you asked influenced your walk, your perception of the walk and how you felt about yourself. Notice how the questions shifted your awareness over time. Write down your observations.

Imagine how these questions can influence you when creating plant medicine or speaking with a client. Write down your thoughts.

Meditation

Walking Meditation – Golden Bones

Go for a quiet walk, by yourself. Walk in a familiar place so you are not concerning yourself with an environment that may presents hazards or uncertainty. Try to pick a place with a clear path that is not too busy. You don't want to be dodging skate boarders and cyclists or patting dogs.

As you walk feel your bones. Begin with your feet. Become aware of how the tiny bones in your feet move with each step.

Then consider the bones in your ankles. Feel them roll against each other as you walk.

Next feel the bones in your lower leg. Open to their strength.

Feel the bones in your knee slide with each step.

Contact the strength in the thigh bone.

Feel the movement of the hip bones as you walk and the extension of the spine.

Notice how your rib cage opens and closes and how the bones in your arms and hands swing with each step.

Notice the weight of your skull.

Now image a gold light shines from within your bones and continue walking.

When you have finished your walk think:

May the peace I have gathered with this short meditation practice be shared with all others so they may be peaceful.

Reflection

First of all the twinkling stars vibrated, but remained motionless in space, then all the celestial globes united into one series of movements... Firmaments and planets both disappeared, but the mighty breath which gives life to all things and which all is bound up remained. – Vincent Van Gogh

A Study of the Elements

Watch the wind move through trees. Then watch the wind move across the water. Listen to the wind in different landscapes. See if you can discern the songs the wind sings as it moves through different trees. Mimic the sounds the wind makes. Study the wind. Study your breath and how it moves through your body.

Understanding Body/Mind

One of the first signs of illness is a lack of movement. Initially only a small part of the body is still. For example: a sluggish bowel, or a stiff neck. As an illness progresses the lack of movement spreads. Lassitude and malaise settle in. Or perhaps pain spreads, which hinders movement. Often people who are extremely ill do not have the strength for movement. With movement they grunt, groan and sigh. Each sound is an expression of stagnancy, a release of breathe.

One could also consider repetitive thinking as a lack of movement. Chronically repetitive thoughts lead to stagnation in life and a lack of creativity.

Movement of the body can help resolve repetitive thoughts. Movement of the body can heal pain. We are built to move.

Physical movement massages our inner organs and keeps the water element flowing in our body. Physical movement wakes up the fire element. As you do the following two exercises see if you can see changes in the water element and fire element in your body. How are the water and fire elements affected by movement?

1. For one week do some kind of movement twice a day. Perhaps you decide to go for a walk and participate in a 20-minute Youtube yoga video. Or perhaps you go for a bike ride and a swim. You may want crank up some music and dance. Change it up. But for one week, move your body for 20 minutes twice a day.

Notice how you feel at the end of the week. Be aware of your both your body and mind.

2. Now do not move for one week. Do not go for a walk, bike ride, dance, yoga, etc....

Notice how you feel at the end of the week. Be aware of both your body and mind.

Creative Plant Monographs

Willow (Salix alba)

Solomon seal (Polygonatum biflorum)

Wild Yam (Dioscorea villosa)

Comfrey (Symphytum spp.)

Celery (Apium graveolens)

Aconite (Aconitium spp)

Enhancing Herbal Knowledge

1. Name three plants that contain allantoin. Why are these plants useful to the herbalist? Describe three ways you can recommend a client take use these plants.

2. Name three plants that contain salicin. Why are these plants useful to the herbalist? Describe how salicin works in the body. How does salicin's action differ from those of aspirin?

3. Name three plants that remove uric acid. Why are these plants useful to the herbalist? How are the kidneys related to the removal of uric acid from the body?

4. Find a protocol for taking Homeopathic Arnica. Why is this protocol important to a herbalist?

5. What recommendations would you make if someone was going to use a tincture of arnica internally?

Medicine Making

Massage Oil

Try making these 4 different massage oils and test them out. Make notes about how each oil works and ways you may want to use the oils for different types of health challenges.

1. In 1/2 cup of peanut oil (peanut oil has anti-inflammatory properties) add 10 drops of wintergreen essential oil. Try the oil out.

2. In ½ cup of peanut oil add 10 drops of ginger essential oil. Try the oil out.

3. In ½ cup of peanut oil add 10 drops of peppermint essential oil. Try the oil out.

4. Now make a massage oil that contains all three essential oils. Try the oil out.

Create a pain cream

The following is a basic cream recipe. Although I dislike cleaning up after making creams (the blender is a challenge to clean) I prefer creams over salves. While salves are generally made with infused oils hardened with beeswax, creams are a combination of oil and water.

Blending water and oil is not always easy. I have failed at making creams many times: the water and oil have separated. But because I can add tinctures and medicinal teas to creams to create strong topical medicine for pain, rashes, basil cell carcinomas, etc., I have persevered and for the most part make a pretty decent cream.

I suggest you begin with making the basic recipe and perfecting it. Then move on to adaptations using tinctures and teas. One caution about teas: make sure you add a preservative in the cream like alcohol from a tincture because the extra bacteria that teas introduce will spoil your medicine quicker than you wish.

The Basic recipe:

In pot combine

¾ cup of oil

1/3 cup of coconut oil

½ to 1 oz of grated beeswax

Heat gently until wax is melted. Do not simmer or boil. Remove from heat.

In the blender combine...

2/3 cup distilled water

1/3 cup aloe vera gel (not juice)

Essential oils of your choice.

When the oils have cooled to the point where they are lukewarm to touch, turn the blender on at a medium speed and slowly pour the oils in.

Blend as well as you can. When the blender is no longer blending, stir with a large spoon.

When you are ready to make a pain cream you can create an infused oil of comfrey or St. John's Wort to add to the oil portion of your cream.

To your water portion, add tinctures of lobelia, cayenne, willow, california poppy, aconite, wild lettuce, etc. I generally put the tinctures in the measuring cup and then once I have added the tincture I fill the cup to the 2/3's mark with water.

There are many essential oils you can use such as: black pepper, ginger, white birch, peppermint, just to name a few.

Be sure to familiarize yourself with these plants (tinctures and essential oils) before you use them.

Record your medicine making in detail when making creams and be sure to give clear instructions on how to use the cream to cause no harm while offering the greatest benefit.

Dreams

Pick a dream symbol and act it out. For example: if you dream of a crow flying, fly like a crow. Of if you dream of a man with a jack hammer, act out the man using a jack hammer. If dream of climbing a ladder, pretend you are climbing a ladder.

As you act out the dream symbol, imagine you are the ambiance of the dream.
Notice how your body responds to acting out the dream symbol. Record your insights.

Lesson Ten:
Dreaming Medicine

Please read chapter ten in *The Herbal Apprentice: Plant Medicine and The Human Being.*

Healer Heal Thyself

As I write this Rufus Wainwright is singing *Somewhere Over the Rainbow*: the sad song of cement feet without hope of flight. It is a song that does not believe anything is possible. Is this true? Can we fly beyond the rainbow?

Notice your response to these questions. Are you thinking, now has she really lost it? Or are you thinking, of course I can fly over the rainbow? If you are thinking either thought, you are absolutely right.

Our minds are very, very big places. We can dream up anything. Just pick up a science fiction novel or watch a horror movie and before you know it off you go on a story (aka dream) that evokes emotions, challenges belief systems, hardens opinions and shifts your reality.

And at the end of it all we know it was just a story. But our experience of the story was real and changed something inside of us. We are never quite the same again even though it was just a story. How does that happen? Does something have to be "real" or "true" to change us?

Our stories and dreams shape us.

Yesterday a man was telling me he was broken. He was broken almost 30 years ago. Then he told me another story about an event that happened before he was born. What else happened in those 30 years I ask him? He was unsure of what to say.

"What do you mean?" he asked. He has forgotten much of his dream.

The other day a woman told me she has been diagnosed with a mental illness. She told me she is finally ready to "deal" with it and asked me if I had any plant medicine that could help her get rid of it. I considered her request and the thought arose that her mental illness was not a rare disease, but self-hatred. So I told her the only treatment I know for self-hatred is love. She gasped and awoke from her dream of self-hatred.

The belief she is wrong, shameful and sick perpetuated her illness and wrapped her in a dream about something unknown that eluded her, a cure or perhaps a reason for her ongoing shame. She dreams every day that there is something wrong with her that must be hidden. This simply is not true, not in my reality of her. Who is right?

Our minds tell powerful stories about identity, possibilities, obstacles and reality. Some of our stories are helpful and some are not. It is important to understand the limit of their truth. Katie Byron, a self-help Guru, encourages people to probe the truth of their stories by asking, "Is this true?"

It is shocking how quickly this question can shatter a dream and enrich life. Try it next time you find yourself caught in an endlessly repeating story.

It's here though that we must be careful. Just because there is always another truth to add to any story or another interpretation to any dream, does not mean we negate the man who feels broken or the woman who is ashamed of a diagnosis. Both carry a truth that needs to be acknowledged and felt. Both stories need to be explored until the heart of compassion shines light on the full truth of their being. Remember the experience of being broken is part of the richness of who they are.

This is a cautionary tale for healers. Often we are tempted to negate the story of suffering because our experience is more than the story being told or we tumble in the dream the illness spins and fail to see the grace in the human being sitting in front of us.

The healer's dream is one that keeps her feet firmly planted on the ground while she flies over the rainbow.

Try this...

1. Three times a day, look around and say to yourself: "This is a dream." Notice how this affects your perception and sense of freedom. Or does it freak you out! If it does, stop the exercise.

2. Travel to a place you have never been. Choose a place that does not seem like it would be a good "fit" for you. For example: if you dislike fast food take a trip to a fast food restaurant, particularly one of the more infamous ones. Notice your perceptions and self-referencing. How do you create an identity around "who you are not." See if you can experience the place like a dream. Try going to a few different places outside of your comfort zone and see what happens. It could be a store you do not frequent, a neighbourhood, even a movie you would never choose. Make notes of your findings.

3. Write how you feel about the people who go to these places outside of your comfort one.

4. Notice a story you tell yourself several times a day or week. It may be about a job, a place, person, or yourself. Then when you find yourself telling the story to yourself, ask, "What else is true?" Record your insights.

5. When someone you know tells you a story that seems well rehearsed, like they have told it a hundred times before, ask them, "What else is true?" Record your insights.

Meditation

Blessing Plants

Human beings have the capacity to bless the environment they pass through. Unfortunately, we are usually so caught in dreams that have nothing to do with the place we are passing through. We lose sight of this miraculous gift we can offer the world. Take some time to bless the world with your presence.

Go for a walk where there are many different types of plants. Preferably some plants you do not know by name. As you walk practice loving-kindness meditation from Lesson One. Gently say to yourself:

May I be well and happy

May I be free from anxiety, disease and anger

May I guard myself with happiness.

Enjoy the feeling of loving-kindness.

When you feel loving-kindness flowing from your heart, touch the plants as you walk by them and wish them happiness.

Be aware of the loving-kindness flowing from your hand and into the plants you touch.

After a while stop actively practicing loving-kindness, sit down and rest.

Feel the loving-kindness of the plants flowing back into you.

(If you can't get a feeling of loving-kindness flowing, just touch the plants and wish them happiness and see what happens.)

Reflection

For there is nothing to guarantee that we will be able to remain long enough or deeply enough in front of the unknown, a psychological state which the traditional paths have always recognized as sacred. In that fleeting state between dreams, which is called "despair" in some Western teachings and "self-questioning" in Eastern traditions, a man is said to be able to receive the truth, both about nature and his own possible role in the universal order. – Jacob Needleman

Understanding the Body/Mind

Note: When doing this practice do not linger in any one area of the body. Offer each area of your body 3 breaths and move on.

The Elements Manifesting in Your Body

The elements will present different textures or feelings in your body. You may want to choose one element to focus on each time you do this exercise.

The water element is experienced as sticky or flowing.
The earth element is experienced as soft or hard.
The fire element is experienced as hot or cold.
The wind element is experienced as vibration.

You will find some areas of your body that are numb. Everyone has numbness. Be curious, don't fret, offer 3 breaths and move on. The numb feeling will evolve.

Lay down on your back on your bed. Leave the lights on so you do not fall asleep.

Take 3 deep breaths and then let your breath settle.

When you feel ready:

Breathe into your left foot. See if you can identify a texture in your left foot. For example: does it feel hard or soft, brittle or thick, tight or loose? If you cannot feel anything in particular notice that and then move on.

Breathe into your right foot. Again try to identify a texture in your right foot.

Carry on in this manner:

Lower left leg, lower right leg.

Upper left leg, upper right leg.

Pelvis

Abdomen

Chest

Left shoulder, right shoulder

Upper left arm, upper right arm

Lower left arm, lower right arm

Left hand, right hand

Neck

Back of head

Face

Rest and count 21 breaths.

And repeat body scan.

Do you notice any emotions contained in any area of your body?

Return to an area of your body that was painful or difficult to feel or just curious to you and ask: *What plant would be good for this area?* See what happens.

Creative Monographs

Mugwort (*Artemisia vulgaris*)

Belladona (*Atropa belladonna*)

Sweet Grass (*Hierochloe odorata*)

White Sage *(Salvia apiana)*

Cannabis (*Cannabis sativa*) (*Cannabis incus*)

Enhancing Herbal Knowledge

Doctrine of Signatures

Create a doctrine of signatures for three plants.

Go for a walk where many plants grow. Preferably ones you do not know well.

As you walk, notice the plants. Bless them. And then ask:

Who is Watching You? (meaning a plant, not a person)

As you walk around you will sense one particular plant's interest in you.

Pause by the plant and look around asking yourself the following questions:

What kind of area is the plant growing in?

What is growing around it?

Is the plant healthy, or does it appear unhealthy?

Jot down answers to these questions in a notebook.

Then sit down next to the plant.

Draw the plant. Focus on different parts of the plant. Don't worry, no one is going to look at your drawing. Do any parts of the plant bring to mind parts of the body or characteristic signs of illness?

The colours of the different parts of the plant often suggest its medicine. What colours are present in the plant?

Touch the plant. Explore its different parts with the tips of your fingers. What does the texture of the plant bring to mind?

Smell the plant — the whole plant. Does the scent of the plant evoke memories?

Taste the plant if you feel it is safe to do so. You can always spit it out. (Herbalists know how to spit.) Is there a physical or mental experience that arises when tasting the plant? Do the flowers taste different from the leaves? The leaves from the stem? The stem from the root?

Practice giving and receiving breathing with the plant by offering your carbon dioxide carried on your breath and receiving the oxygen the plant exhales.

When you feel quiet inside, mentally ask the plant:

How can I help you?

Then ask:

How can you help me?

Jot down notes on your conversation in your notebook.

Hypothesize about the medicine the plant carries.

When you return home do book research on the plant.

Where does your intuitive and analytic understanding of the plants meet?

Medicine Making

Make a Dream Sachet

In a small sachet add the following herbs: Mugwort, hops and lavender. You can play with the portions of each herb in the sachet to best suit the medicine you wish the dream sachet to offer. For example: if you want more dreams, use more Mugwort. If you want more calm, use more lavender. If you need deeper sleep, try adding more hops.

Place your dream sachet inside your pillowcase. Notice the difference.

If you forget to take the dream sachet out of the pillowcase when you launder your bedding, your sheets will be scented with lavender.

Create a Smudge

All traditions of plant medicine use smoke medicine. I find smoke medicine endlessly fascinating! I know one Cree herbalist who says he relieved the hallucinations of a schizophrenic using a smudge mixture. He believes that smudging can ease most mental illness.

When I lived on the prairie and in the Yukon, I often used buffalo sage (*Artemisia frigida*) in my smudge mixtures as it was easily available near the places that I lived. Where I live now, it is not so hard to find. Buffalo sage is burnt to purify. Just before we left the Yukon we found ourselves living in a house full of ghosts. We burnt large amounts of Buffalo sage and made many, many prayers to allow the ghosts to move on. When we left the house, the atmosphere was sparkling with light.

Last summer, I planted a large patch of sweetgrass and hope to be able to gather it in a couple of years to make as smoke medicine. Sweetgrass smoke brings peace.

Most aromatic herbs can be used in a smudge. The Artemsia family are traditional smudge plants that are easy to find. Often I use Mugwort as my primary plant in the smudge and then add smaller amounts of aromatic herbs. Three of my favorites are lavender, rosemary and rose petals.

Create your own smudge. Explore different combinations of aromatic plants. Sit quietly when you burn them. Notice how the smudge makes you feel. How it changes the atmosphere in the room.

Always, make good notes.

Dreams

Finding Your Inner Herbalist

On a beautiful piece of paper, by hand, write a letter introducing yourself to your inner herbalist. You do not yet know your inner herbalist's name. That is okay. This is a letter to begin to make a connection with the part of you that understands plant medicine and how to use it to help others with complete confidence. You are a student, so of course you do not feel this way.

In your letter ask your inner herbalist for help in understanding plant medicine. You may want to ask the herbalist what his or her name is. Describe the type of relationship you hope to form with your inner herbalist. Write to your inner herbalist about the type of herbalist you want to become. Tell the herbalist why you feel herbal medicine is important. Ask for guidance.

When you have finished writing the letter, put in under your pillow. Each night as you fall asleep ask for a dream from your inner herbalist. Do this for 3 nights. If you do not receive a dream, wait 3 days, write another letter, put it under your pillow and ask for another dream.

Record your dream in the form of a letter from your inner herbalist. The letter may not be like the dream.

Lesson Eleven
Medicine Making: The Art of Opportunists

Please read chapter eleven in The Herbal Apprentice: Plant Medicine and The Human Being.

Healer Heal Thyself

Bears are the totem animal of herbalists. Some say it is because they have a keen sense of the medicine contained in roots. For example, the bears that live on the wind side of the Rocky Mountains have a deep understanding of Osha's (*Ligusticum porter*) medicine areas. The first ritual a bear performs upon waking from hibernation is digging up Osha roots. The bear chews, mixing it with saliva (saliva is an excellent solvent for plant medicine as the enzymes it contains breaks down cell walls), until it's a slimy paste. The bear then squirts this medicine rich in volatile oils and saponins all over its body, rolls around on the ground and rubs it into its fur. Osha is a strong anti-microbial and anti-parasitic. You can just image all the life that has taken up lodgings on the bear sleeping for several cold months in a mound of old leaves and dirt. Once clean, the male bears take roots to female bears and perform the same ritual for her before spring mating.

I do not question the bear's understanding of plant medicine, however, the great gift a bear shows herbalists is their opportunist tendencies. Another way to say this is: "Don't believe everything you read and only stick with that knowledge."

It is early spring as I write this piece. My husband and I went forest bathing the other day in Gatineau Park. The water was everywhere, trickling down hillsides, rushing under bridges, overflowing into meadows, pooling on muddy paths. The trees were drinking deeply after their long winter sleep.

This area of the world is famous for its majestic white pines (Pinus strobus). White pines are towering trees, with long sweeping branches and soft tips, even though their needles are sharp. The wind sings gently as it blows through white pines.

The medicine white pine offers is strongly antiseptic with powerful volatile oil. The commonly gathered parts of the tree are its young needles, inner bark, resin and roots. Traditionally all these various parts of the tree are used in remedies to relieve colds, ?, and bronchitis. The needles, high in Vitamin C, are made into teas for colds. A salve is made from the pitch to warm a congested chest. The inner bark is a traditional survival food.

When I was walking in the forest the other day, it was too early to collect the new shoots from the tips of the pine branches. I was not seeing a significant amount of resin flowing from the trees and besides I was in a provincial park where it is illegal to gather plant medicine. I did, like a bear, take an opportunity to gather some white pine medicine.

As I walked I picked up a small branch from a white pine that had fallen in a recent wind storm. On the tips of the branch I found green/purple young pine cones sticky with resin. I plucked it from the branch and popped it in my mouth, using my tongue to access the medicine. My head cleared (I didn't realize how foggy I was) and my sinuses burst open. The hundred scents of spring flooded my brain. I had just discovered medicine.

Unfortunately, it was the only branch with a few young pine cones on it in the area. I put the five cones in my pocket and my husband and I nibbled on them as we walked.

When we returned to the car, I walked over to the outhouse and just to the side of the outhouse someone had pruned several white pines leaving behind huge branches covered with young pine cones. One by one, I plucked them until my pockets were bursting with the cones.

On our way home we picked up a bottle of 94% alcohol, as a high percentage of alcohol is needed to extract resin.

Now the cones are macerating in a jar and I have great medicine to offer to those suffering with bronchitis, sinusitis, colds and chronic phlegmy coughs.

Bears use what they find. What is available to them at the moment. I recommend as a herbalist you take the bears' lead and learn to use what you have available.

Try this...

Consider something you would really like to do that you do not have the resources for. Try not to go BIG with this — do not, for instance, decide you want to live in a 50 room mansion or travel around the world in your private jet — go with something that you have wanted to do for a long time and just have not yet done.

Write the down the reasons for not doing what you desire.

Go through those reasons and edit them. Differentiate between the reasons that are practical and the reasons that are excuses. Cross out the excuses.

Brainstorm possible solutions to the practical causes for you not doing what you wish to do.

Now put a plan into place for doing what you wish and follow the plan to the best of your ability. Watch for opportunities to present themselves.

Meditation

Meditation is a form of medicine making. Meditation, when done with the aspiration to benefit others, turns our lives into medicine for others.

There are many different forms of meditation using the breath that lifts our spirits, quiets our minds and wakes our energy. When making medicine, it is advisable to use these simple practices to help focus you while working with the plants. Try the medicine of Alternate Nostril Breathing as a short meditation to prepare for medicine making.

Alternate Nostril Breathing

1. Sit in a comfortable position with your back straight and let your breath settle.

2. Using your right ring finger gently close your left nostril and slowly inhale through your left nostril.

3. Close off your left nostril with your thumb and slowly exhale from your right nostril.

4. When you are breathing evenly through both nostrils, add this next step:

5. Image that each in breath moves deep into your belly and settles at your navel chakra. The navel chakra is approximately three fingers widths below your navel just in front of your spine.

6. Hold each in breath in the navel chakra for the count of five.

7. Exhale out the alternate nostril.

8. Try to do this 3 times or 7 times or 21 times. As you become more familiar with alternate nostril breathing let your breath become slower and pause for longer periods of time in the navel chakra.

Reflection

I said to my soul, be still, and wait

without hope,

For hope would be hope of the

wrong things. – T.S. Elliot

Understanding Body/Mind

Medicine making is all about chemistry. Mind/Bodies are all about chemistry. Write a page about the following products of chemical interactions in the body. Note the role each plays in our health and how changes in their activity affects our well-being.

Glucose

Adenosine Tri-Phosphate

Iron

Enzymes (a general class of molecules)

Trigylcerides

Water

Creative Monographs

Each of the plants in this section of Creative Monographs can be made into many forms of medicine. Try to discover different ways to make medicine with each plant.

Calendula (Calendula officinalis)

Pine   (Pinus stobus)

Echinacea (Echinacea agustifolia)

Garlic   (Allium sativa)

Plantain (Plantago spp.)

Enhancing Herbal Knowledge

Discover whether the following classes of phytochemicals are water or fat soluble.

If a class of phytochemical is fat soluble, record the percentage of alcohol needed to extract it from the plant.

Inulin

Flavonoids

Terpenoids

Tannins

Saponins

Medicine Making

Tinctures

Tinctures are easy to make if you know what phytochemicals you want to extract from the plant and how to do it. There are also a few tips that will make your tinctures strong efficient medicine.

❖ Try not to purchase powdered herbs. Powdered herbs lose their potency quicker than cut and shifted herbs (c/s) and they are easier to adulterate for the dishonest herb broker.

❖ Powder most of your herbs you plan to tincture. A coffee grinder works well.

Note: if a plant is high in sugars, don't powder.

❖ Try macerating your tincture for different periods of time. I often find macerations of 3 days with frequent shaking makes stronger medicine than macerating plants for longer periods of time.

❖ Let your tincture drip through a coffee filter before you press the remaining mark.

❖ Label! On each tincture you make you need to record the following:

o Botanical name of the plant

o Percentage of alcohol and/or other solvents you use. (You do not need to record the amount of water in the tincture.)

o Ratio of plant to solvent

  ○ Date bottled

 ❖ Remember to keep good medicine making notes.

Make the following tinctures.

You do not need to make a lot of each tincture. Through this exercise I want you to understand how changing the percentage of alcohol to water effects the medicine extracted from the plant and therefore how you use the tincture to help another.

Calendula officinalis 1:4 25%

Calendula officinalis 1:4 40%

Calendula officinalis 1:4 60%

Calendula officinalis 1:3 75%

Dreams

Sit quietly and consider the dream work you have done.

Appendix 1

Herbal Actions

Herbal actions are part essential information and part injustice to wide ranging application of any one herb to support the health of the body. Talking about herbs in terms of actions is like saying all plumbers do emergency house calls, all acupunctures can work on animals and human beings and that all doctors are pill pushes and all herbalists work holistically.

Now that being said, knowing an herb's action is certainly useful when talking about herbal medicine and attempting to convey the therapeutics of a plant. Exploring an herb's actions is a bit like exploring a dream. There are layers to herbal actions that need to be unearthed is one seeks true understanding.

Let's begin with a short quote from Matthew Wood who has thought a great deal about this topic, as part of the language of herbal medicine. *In traditional Western medicine the actions of medicinal plants are described according to three basic classes: physiological imbalances, physiological function, and organ affinity. - The Practice of Traditional Western Herbalism, Matthew Wood pg59*

When we read that an herb is a hepatic, that is an herb with an affinity for the liver. The action of a hepatic is just that. It does not describe an herb that cleanses the liver, not protects the liver. The same is true for nervines, plants with an affinity for the nervous system, pectoral, medicine for the lungs and so on.

A chologue is an herbal action that has an effect on the liver. It increases the secretion on bile from the liver. A diuretic, increases urination, an anti-hypertensive decreases blood pressure, a diaphoretic encourages sweating, and so on. These are herbs that affect physiological function.

An herbalist offers stimulants to offset a physiological imbalance. Relaxants, astringents and demulcents are also herbal actions that provide the body with an action it is lacking.

This is the first layer of understanding an herb action.

An herb's actions will also suggest its chemical make-up and energetics or quality. To understand the activity of an herb, it is important for an herbalist to be able to decipher these two seemingly separate languages of herbal medicine conveyed by an herb's single action.

Some herbals actions are so vague, they are almost meaningless. For example, saying an herb is an anti-inflammatory conveys very little information about the herbs actual action. This is where a student of herbal medicine must dig deeper into the herbs energetics and chemistry.

With all this in mind, study the following chart in order to begin to discover the language of herbal medicine. Please note, among herbalists these terms can take on different meanings. Confused? No worries, over time it all comes together.

Action: Adaptogen
Class: Physiological function
Action in the body: Modulates the activity of the adrenal glands
Chemistry: Frequently saponins which mimic hormone precursors
Energetics: Herb specific
Examples: Eleuthrococcus, Ashwagndha, Panax ginseng, Licorice, Rhodiola
Notes: These are generally tonic herb which taken over a period of time affect every part of the body.

Action: Alterative
Class: Physiological function
Action in the body: Cleansing and often nourishing
Chemistry: Herb specific
Energetics: Herb specific
Examples: Burdock, black walnut husks, echinacea, red clover, nettles, yellow doc, garlic
Notes: These plants are traditionally referred to as blood cleansers. They have overall diverse actions on the body and each asks that it is understood on its own terms.

Action: Anti-microbial
Class: Physiological imbalance
Action in the body: Kills pathogens
Chemistry: Volatile oils, resins and alkaloids
Energetics: Plant specific

Examples: Barberry, myrrh, garlic, thyme
Notes: This action includes yeast, virus' and bacteria, parasites.

Action: Antispasmodics or spasmolytic
Class: Physiological function
Action in the body: Calms spasms within smooth muscle tissue.
Chemistry: Volatile oils and alkaloids are frequently found but because this is a wide ranging activity, there are many ways a plant calms muscle tension.
Energetics: Cooling or warming
Examples: Hops, ginger, parsley, lobelia, black cohosh
Notes: Antispasmodics in the GI tract are called carminatives

Action: Astringents
Class: Physiological imbalance
Action in the body: Acts on membranes and skin
Chemistry: Tannins
Energetics: Drying
Examples: Blackberry leaf, agrimony, raspberry, plantain, sage
Notes: Different astringents have different organ affinities, for example blackberry is specific to the colon whereas sage acts more on the respiratory tract

Action: Bitter
Class: Physiological function
Action in the body: Stimulates the parasympathetic system and bile secretion.
Chemistry: Herb specific
Energetics: Generally cooling however often when combined with volatile oil the bitter is overpowered and the plant is warming.
Examples: Strongest: Gentian and wormwood Mild: Chamomile Bitter/pungent: Elecampane
Notes: Traditional remedies for depression and migraine

Cardio- tonic
Class: Organ specific
Action in the body: Effects the heart
Chemistry: Herb specific, often high in flavonoids
Energetics: Herb specific
Examples: Hawthorn berry, leaf, flower, Linden flowers, Motherwort
Notes: Cardio-tonics can also be classed as hypotensive although this is a more physiological effect. I tend to separate the two actions out.

Action: Carminatives
Class: Physiological function
Action in the body: Calms spasms in the gut
Chemistry: Volatile oils
Energetics: Warming (generally)
Examples: Ginger, peppermint, melissa
Notes: Melissa and chamomile are two carminative which are considered cooling

Action: Circulatory Stimulants
Class: Physiological function
Action in the body: Enhances circulation.
Chemistry: Herb specific
Energetics: Warming and can be drying
Examples: Cayenne, ginger, prickly ash, rosemary
Notes: Specific circulatory stimulants have a more pronounced effect on different parts of the body.

Action: Cholagogue
Class: Physiological function
Action in the body: Stimulate bile flow from the liver (often bitter flavor)
Chemistry: Herb specific
Energetics: Herb specific
Examples: Dandelion root, sage leaf, yellow doc, wild yam, artichoke leaf, melissa

Notes: Because these herbs increase bile flow, they support the body in digesting fat and have a laxative effect, therefore they are cleansing for the whole body. These herbs are contra-indicated when there is sever distress in the liver or gallbladder.

Action: Demulcent
Class: Physiological imbalance
Action in the body: Moistens and soothes mucous membranes
Chemistry: Mucilage
Energetics: Cooling and moist
Examples: Marshmallow, comfrey, calendula (calendula is warmer than most demulcents)
Notes: When used internally herb with mucilage are called demulcents, externally vulnerary

Action: Diuretics
Class: Physiological function
Action in the body: Stimulates urination
Chemistry: Various, many of these plants have volatile oils that irritate the kidney into voiding. Others are high in minerals that stimulate voiding through altered electrolyte balance.
Energetics: Plants high in volatile oils are generally warming.
Plants high in minerals are generally cooling. Think of heat leaving the body with the urine.
Examples: Plants high in volatile oils: juniper, yarrow. Parsley. Plants high in minerals: dandelion leaf, parsley, nettle
Notes: Loosely speaking, many use the term diuretic to define an herb that acts on the kidney and does not necessary increase urination.
Note: herbs that act on the cardiovascular system often have influence on the kidney.

Action: Emollient
Class: Physiological imbalance
Action in the body: Softens dry skin
Chemistry: Oils or mucilage
Energetics: Cooling and moist

Examples: Cocoa butter, aloe vera, strawberry
Notes: Emollients are used specifically on the skin.

Action: Emmenagogue
Class: Physiological function
Action in the body: Stimulates the uterus to shed the endometrium
Chemistry: Various: alkaloids in some cases
Energetics: Herb specific
Examples: Motherwort, black cohosh, blue cohosh, Mugwort
Notes: Today's herbalists often use the term emmenagogue to define an herb that acts on the uterus. Under this definition Raspberry would be considered an emmenagogue. Because, emmenagogue are contra-indicated in the first two semesters of pregnancy, I recommend differentiating between uterine tonics and emmenagogue. In this case, raspberry would be an uterine tonic.

Action: Expectorant
Class: Physiological function
Action in the body: Stimulate the cough reflex or creates a productive cough.
Chemistry: Volatile oils, alkaloids, saponins and mucilage are all found in expectorants.
Energetics: Stimulating expectorants are warming and drying. Relaxing expectorants are moistening and generally cooling
Examples: Stimulating expectorants: Thyme, elecampane, Osha Relaxing expectorants: licorice, marshmallow, hyssops
Notes: Stimulating expectorants are used in productive coughs. Relaxing expectorants are used in a dry cough.

Action: Hepatic
Class: Organ specific
Action in the body: Protects the liver
Chemistry: herb specific
Energetics: herb specific but often cooling
Examples: Milk Thistle, schisandra, rosemary, globe artichoke

Notes: These plants are not necessarily used for detoxification

Action: Immune modulating
Class: Organ specific
Activity in the body: Brings balance to the immune system
Chemistry: Herb specific (often polysaachrides)
Energetics: Herb specific
Examples: Astragulus, ashwagandha, echinacea
Notes: These herbs do not necessarily stimulate the immune system, and are often used in auto-immune conditions

Action: Laxative
Class: Physiological function
Action in the body: Stimulate peristalsis in the bowel resulting in bowel movements. Specifically used in cases of constipation.
Chemistry: Although not all many contain anthroquiones
These constituents irritate the bowel wall initiating peristalsis. The more irritating the laxative, more sever the cramping will be.
Energetics: Herb specific
Examples: Mild: Yellow doc, oregon grape root, licorice, flax seed Mild to strong: Turkey rhubarb Strong: Senna, cascara
Notes: Laxatives are classes according to there effects: cathartics are violent and quick in action and often result in watery stool. *Purgatives* produce semi-solid stool and are more powerful than laxatives. Actual laxatives are gentler in their action. These herbs are often combined with carminatives.

Action: Lymphatic
Class: Organ specific
Action in the body: Effects the lymphatic system
Chemistry: Herb specific
Energetics: Herb specific
Examples: Red clover, cleavers, wild violet leaf, echinacea
Notes: These herbs can be confused with alteratives, because they are usually also alterative. The class of herbs called alteratives tend to have

a wider range of actions.

Action: Nephritic
Class: Organ specific
Action in the body: Protects the kidneys and urinary tract
Chemistry: herb specific
Energetics: herb specific
Examples: Goldenrod, parsley piert,
Notes: This action is frequent confused with diuretics, which effect physiological function.

Nervine
Class: Organ specific
Action in the body: Effects the nervous system
Chemistry: Varies, can be high mineral content in plant, volatile oils or the complex chemistry of an individual plant.
Energetics: Herb specific
Examples: Tonics: Wild oats, skullcap, St John's Wort.
Notes: One can divide nervines into more specific actions: relaxant, stimulant, hypnotic, anti-spasmodic, anti-depressant, adaptogen, analgesic.

Action: Pectorals
Class: Organ specific
Action in the body: Protects the lungs and bronchi
Chemistry: herb specific
Energetics: herb specific
Examples: Licorice, astragulus, schisandra
Notes: This action is frequent confused with expectorants, which effect physiological function

Action: Sedatives
Class: Physiological function
Action in the body: Used to induce calm or sleep

Chemistry: Volatile oils and alkaloids are frequently found but because this is a wide ranging activity, there are many ways a plant sedates activity.

Energetics: Cooling

Examples: Valerian (warming in nature), hops, passionflower, california poppy

Notes: Sedative herbs are dose specific, one can use lower doses to relax without sedating. If working with insomnia, be sure you have the big picture, before offering sedatives. These herbs are also referred to as hypnotics.

Action: Stimulants

Class: Physiological function

Action in the body: Stimulate a specific organs activity

Chemistry: Volatile oils and alkaloids are frequently found but because this is a wide ranging activity, there are many ways a plant stimulates activity.

Energetics: Warming

Examples: Coffee, rosemary, cayenne, panax ginseng

Notes: Stimulants tend to have an organ affinity, for example turkey rhubarb's laxative effect is stimulating to the bowel whereas thyme stimulates the cough reflex

Action: Styptics

Class: Physiological function

Action in the body: Slows bleeding, both external and internal

Chemistry: Herb specific, often tannins

Energetics: Dry

Examples: Shepard's Purse, Yarrow, Cayenne, Nettles

Notes: These herbs are generally offered in frequent low doses until bleeding stops.

Appendix Two

Herbs and Medicine Making Supplies You'll Need

Lesson	Herbs	Other Supplies
Lesson #1	Hawthorn Berries (Wild craft if possible) Rosehips (Wild craft if possible)	Sachet Honey Cheese clothe Distilled water
Lesson #2	Rosemary, Tea Tree and Lavender essential oils Fresh ginger Fresh garlic Thyme Garlic	Honey Apples Large pickle jar Orange
Lesson #3	Peppermint Lemon balm Fresh Ginger Caraway Seeds Fennel Seeds Rosemary	Apple cider vinegar Honey Cabbage Salt
Lesson #4	Rosemary	Castor oil Distilled water
Lesson #5	Sage Thyme Astragulus root Cinnamon Rosemary	A whole chicken Apple cider vinegar Garlic Onion Wine (red or white) Prunes Thompson raisons Dried figs

		Dried apricots
		3 Apples
		2 Pears
		Molasses
Lesson #7	Poplar buds (Wild craft if possible) Calendula flowers (Grow and dry if possible)	Oat flakes (Not instant)
Lesson #8	Dill Your choice of herbs	Grapeseed oil
Lesson #9	Essential oils: Peppermint, sweet birch, ginger	Coconut oil Beeswax Aleo vera gel (not juice) Peanut oil
Lesson #10	Mugwort Hops Lavendar	Sachet
Lesson #11	Calendula flowers	40% alcohol Vodka 95% Alcohol

Appendix Three

Reading List

The Herbal Apprentice: Plant Medicine and the Human Being

By Abrah Arneson

Bartram's Herbal Medicine Encyclopedia

By Thomas Bartram

Holistic Herbal: A Safe and Practical Guide to Making and Using Herbal Remedies
By David Hoffman

The Lost Language of Plants

By Stephen Harrod Buhner

Medicinal Plants of The Pacific West

By Michael Moore

Rosemary Gladstar's Herbal Recipes for Vibrant Health:

175 Teas, Tonics, Oils, Salves, Tinctures,

and Other Natural Remedies for the Entire Family

By Rosemary Gladstar

The Book of Herbal Wisdom

By Matthew Wood

The Anatomy Colouring Book

By Wynn Kapit

Holistic Anatomy: An Integrative Guide to The Human Body

By Pip Waller

Healing Plants of The Rocky Mountains

By Darcy Williamson

About the Author

Abrah Arneson's personal journey began with a life threatening illness that found her on life supports for 6 weeks in an intensive care unit. This experience was her first step in her education towards holistic plant based medicine.

Abrah lived in a meditation retreat centre for eight year studying the relationship between the body, mind and the environment (which includes water, air, forests, gardens and other people). She is a graduate of Dominion Herbal College four-year Clinical Herbal Therapist Diploma Program in Burnaby, British Columbia. Abrah spend seven years working in palliative care and is trained as a doula. Abrah has been a practicing Clinical Herbalist for 10 years.

Abrah has training in iridology, Bach Flower essences and is a Reiki Master. Abrah is author of The Herbal Apprentice: Plant Medicine and the Human Being.

Made in the USA
Middletown, DE
26 March 2023

27697219R00076